ANAESTHETICS FOR
MEDICAL STUDENTS

He that shortens the road to knowledge lengthens life.

Lacon, C. C. Colton.

ANAESTHETICS FOR MEDICAL STUDENTS

GORDON OSTLERE

M.A., M.B., B.Chir.(Camb.), D.A., F.F.A.R.C.S.

Formerly
Deputy First Assistant, Nuffield Department of
Anaesthetics, University of Oxford

ROGER BRYCE-SMITH

M.A., D.M.(Oxon.), D.A., F.F.A.R.C.S.

Formerly
Consultant Anaesthetist, United Oxford Hospitals
Lecturer in Anaesthetics, University of Oxford
Assistant Professor of Anaesthesia, Western Reserve
University, Cleveland, Ohio

With a Foreword by

C. LANGTON HEWER

M.B., B.S., M.R.C.P., F.F.A.R.C.S.
Consulting Anaesthetist, St. Bartholomew's Hospital

NINTH EDITION

CHURCHILL LIVINGSTONE
EDINBURGH LONDON MELBOURNE AND NEW YORK
1980

CHURCHILL LIVINGSTONE
Medical Division of Longman Group UK Limited

Distributed in the United States of America by Churchill
Livingstone Inc., 1560 Broadway, New York, N.Y.
10036 and by associated companies, branches and
representatives throughout the world.

First Edition 1949
Second Edition 1951
Third Edition 1956
Fourth Edition 1960
Fifth Edition 1963
Sixth Edition 1966
Seventh Edition 1972
Eighth Edition 1976
Ninth Edition 1980
    Reprinted 1982
    Reprinted 1984
    Reprinted 1986 (twice)

ISBN 0-443-01863-4

British Library Cataloguing in Publication Data

Ostlere, Gordon
    Anaesthetics for medical students. — 9th ed.
    1. Anaesthesia
    I. Title   II. Bryce-Smith, Roger
    617'.96   RD81   80-40602

Produced by Longman Singapore Publishers Pte Ltd
Printed in Singapore

FOREWORD TO THE FIRST EDITION

There are in existence a large number of textbooks on anaesthesia, some of great merit, but none really caters for the needs of the undergraduate anaesthetic clerk.

This unfortunate individual is in process of acquiring and retaining (until his final examinations) a huge assortment of facts and theories, and the short time that he can spare for anaesthesia must be essentially practical.

Dr Ostlere does not fall into the common error of attempting to explain the scientific reasons for all the phenomena of anaesthesia. This may be the most desirable approach from the educational aspect, but the student simply has not got the time for it. If he can give a straightforward anaesthetic safely for the common operations he has made excellent use of his appointment, and this book should help him to do so.

Some critics may carp at the somewhat colloquial style of the author. It is true that not all the periods are Johnsonian in character, but surely this is a good fault. It is all very well to describe the prognosis of delayed chloroform poisoning as "the pathological changes and metabolic dysfunction are not infrequently so advanced as to become irreversible", but the student is much more likely to remember the gravity of the condition if he reads that "it is usually fatal".

Most textbooks are intolerably dull: this one is frequently amusing and for this reason alone should prove popular.

London, 1949   C. Langton Hewer

PREFACE

This book was written in Auckland harbour during a dock strike in the New Zealand winter of 1948. Dr Bryce-Smith has stringently revised the text since the third edition, the original author being responsible for the editorial work.

Anaesthetics for medical students today is a theoretical more than a practical study. But it affords the student some insight into the specialist anaesthetist's problems and — more valuably — experience in the management of the unconscious patient. The basic principles have not changed since the first edition, and we hope this book will continue to lighten the student's difficulties in the operating theatre and the examination room. We ask him to bear in mind, as we have, that the book circulates in that large area of our world where medicine is practiced less elaborately, and where he may one day possibly find himself.

The size is much the same, so that it may still be studied between theatre cases, on the bus, or while awaiting the entrance of an unpunctual surgeon. We can only hope that nothing has painfully dated except the jokes. This is the last edition in our hands.

Gordon Ostlere
Roger Bryce-Smith

London and Oxford 1980

CONTENTS

CONTENTS

CHAPTER 1
Introductory

Please may we make it clear to you that this small book—which will not take you more than a couple of evenings to devour—is mainly about *General Anaesthetics*. Although there are two types of anaesthetics:

> General
> Local (which includes spinal),

general anaesthesia is the form most frequently practised in this country, and it is adaptable to the greatest number of surgical procedures. In these days of specialization the opportunities for you occasionally to turn anaesthetist are few, but entering general practice will make you liable to give an anaesthetic throughout your professional lifetime for such procedures as forceps delivery, incision of abscess, or manipulation. In any case, it is your duty to know what anaesthesia entails, and to be able to answer the questions of your patients, even though the practice of anaesthesia remains far from your ambitions. We also have in mind the medical missionary who must of necessity turn his hand to anything[1] and our colleagues who work in less favoured parts of the world.

The purpose of this book is to give you an introduction to the subject and, at a pinch, to encourage you to follow the simplest methods of anaesthesia. These may not be the ideal ones, but at least they are safe and reasonably sure. By becoming familiar with these techniques you will have something to fall back on after qualification if you are obliged to give an anaesthetic. By limiting your repertoire and placing an

---

[1] A general practitioner of our acquaintance left his group practice for six months' work in a mission hospital. For several months beforehand he revised his knowledge of anaesthetics, so that on arrival he was not too put out to be informed that a Caesarean Section was imminent. He was less happy to discover that all the other doctors on the station had gone on leave and that he had to operate as well. Mother and baby survived, memorials to what you can do when you really have to.

1

emphasis on safety, you will save yourself many moments of mental discomfort. We are not concerned with the specialized techniques required by thoracic or neurosurgeons, but neither will you be.

Your problems should be fairly straightforward, and it is not too difficult to give a safe and satisfactory anaesthetic if you remember to

(1) Work within the limits of your ability — don't try any fancy tricks witnessed from the experts.

(2) Keep your head in all emergencies.[1]

(3) Remember — safety first. Anaesthetics are dangerous drugs and it is not at all difficult for carelessness to lead to a death on the table. Even though you may not aspire to being an expert anaesthetist you must at least become a safe one. So let us re-apply the maternal advice: If you can't be good, be careful.

(4) Finally, bear in mind that you can learn to give anaesthetics only in the operating theatre, and the more administrations you perform under supervision while unqualified the more you will later appreciate your conscientiousness.

Although most students seem to expect their textbooks to begin by telling them exactly how to give an anaesthetic, the process cannot be explained before considering the properties of the agents at our disposal, the apparatus with which they are given, and the signs they produce in the patient. In addition, something must be known of the physiology of anaesthesia, and in particular the student is requested to recall essentials of the physiology of respiration and the circulation, or at least to

[1] The importance of this quality is strikingly illustrated by the story of a London anaesthetist who, obviously deservedly, rose to the head of his profession. He was administering an anaesthetic to a young lady for a dental extraction one insupportably hot afternoon in August. The operation was in the surgery of a fashionable Harley Street dentist and the only onlooker was the young lady's mother, who insisted on staying in the room. The anaesthetist had just established surgical anaesthesia when he was horrified to see the dentist drop at the foot of the chair, overcome by the heat. The mother thought the dentist was dead, screamed, and fainted herself. The anaesthetist was therefore presented within a few seconds with not one unconscious patient but three. What should he do? Displaying the coolness of a confident administrator he promptly picked up a pair of dental forceps, removed the diseased tooth, turned off the anaesthetic, took his wet sponge and revived the dentist by pressing it on his neck, and brought round the mother by throwing the glass of antiseptic mouthwash over her face. He then put on his hat and left the trio to sort it out for themselves.

refresh his memory with the diagram of the regulation of respiration in a textbook of physiology.

Administration of Anaesthetic Drugs

General anaesthetics may be introduced into the body by four different routes. No matter which route is chosen the drug eventually reaches the final common pathway — the circulation. Thus, although there may be differences in the rate of action, a drug will have the same ultimate effect on the body whether it is given orally, rectally, intravenously, or by inhalation.

(1) **By absorption from the stomach.** Used infrequently, usually only with children, for the introduction of premedicant drugs to produce sedation or even unconsciousness in bed before removal to the anaesthetic room.

Advantages
(i) A simple and pleasant way of inducing narcosis.
(ii) An overdose may be reclaimed by a stomach wash-out.

Disadvantages
(i) Difficulty in persuading some children to swallow medicine, which in any case may be vomited.
(ii) Uncertainty of the rate or completeness of absorption from the stomach, particularly when the normal absorptive process is deranged by the thought of a coming operation.
(iii) Ideally, the dose should be previously judged in terms of body weight.

(2) **By absorption from the rectum.** Used for the administration of thiopentone[1] (Pentothal), particularly in children (see p. 48).

Advantages
(i) Useful in children for producing narcosis in bed, particularly in those who must undergo repeated diagnostic procedures, instead of a more frightening form of general anaesthesia.

---

[1] Medical students vary enormously in knowing either official or proprietary names for drugs, but never the two together. We have called all drugs by their proper names, adding the common proprietary one in brackets *when first described*.

(ii) Absorption is more predictable and certain than from the stomach.

Disadvantages
(i) To some children this is an unpleasant way of receiving an anaesthetic.
(ii) The dose must be previously judged in terms of body weight.
(iii) The fluid may be the equivalent of an enema and may be "returned", leaving an unknown quantity within the bowel to be absorbed.

(3) **By direct injection into a vein.** Used frequently, especially for anaesthesia with the ultra-short-acting barbiturates, e.g., thiopentone.

Advantages
(i) Induction may be accomplished with the least discomfort for the patient.
(ii) The most effective means of administering thiopentone.
(iii) The action of the anaesthetic is rapid, as the absorption mechanism of the body is by-passed.
(iv) The minimum of apparatus is required.

Disadvantages
(i) There is no means whatever of withdrawing an overdose, and the action of the drug may be too rapid for the inexperienced to realize an overdose has been given.
(ii) It is dangerously easy to give.
(iii) Difficulty of entering a suitable vein on occasion.
(iv) The danger of tissue damage if the injection is made extravenously.
(v) The likelihood of causing respiratory and/or circulatory depression. The anaesthetist always must be prepared and equipped to combat this when giving an intravenous anaesthetic.

(4) **By absorption from the lungs.** The most frequently used route.

Advantages
(i) The only route possible for most general anaesthetics, which are either gases or vapours.
(ii) Safety. The absorptive mechanism is reliable but not

dangerously rapid, and an overdose can be recovered by (a) washing out the anaesthetic still in the bronchial tree with air or oxygen; (b) allowing the drug already absorbed to be excreted back into the lungs by artificial respiration with air or oxygen.

Disadvantages

(i) The patient may suffer discomfort if the induction of anaesthesia is performed by this route.

(ii) The vapours of volatile anaesthetics are irritant to a varying degree.

(iii) The lungs themselves may be the seat of disease.

(iv) The lungs must continue their normal function completely unimpaired during the administration.

Simple Outline of the Physiology of Anaesthesia

Once an anaesthetic has reached the blood stream it circulates to all the organs in the body. Fortunately, the only structure upon which the drug is required to exert its action, the central nervous system, receives a greater proportion of anaesthetic than any other. This is because (i) the blood supply to the central nervous system is richer than that of any other organ; and (ii) the anaesthetics are all fat-soluble drugs, dissolving readily in a structure of such high fat content.

An anaesthetic inhaled into the lungs is absorbed through the alveolar membrane into the blood stream, as long as the partial pressure of anaesthetic in the blood remains at a lower level than that in the lungs. Anaesthetic carried in the blood stream will similarly become absorbed by the tissues while they, in turn, remain under a lower tension of the drug than the blood. When the administration of the anaesthetic is stopped the process is thrown into reverse: the drug is excreted from the tissues into the blood stream and from the blood stream to the alveoli. The anaesthetic drugs are, of course, absorbed by the other organs of the body, in a direct ratio to their fat content. As expected, the liver absorbs an amount of anaesthetic second to the central nervous system, and the muscles, with their low proportion of fat, take up little of the agents from the circulation. The gases are carried in the blood in simple solution and do not form compounds with haemoglobin.

Many factors are involved in the rate of uptake of an anaesthetic from the lungs, and its excretion. The potency of the agent, the concentration inhaled, the efficiency of the patient's ventilation and circulation are obvious ones. But we meet an apparent anomaly over the solubility of the drug in blood. The relatively insoluble agents such as nitrous oxide produce anaesthesia quickly, while the soluble ones such as ether work slowly. This is because the alveolar concentration of an insoluble anaesthetic comes rapidly in equilibrium with the inhaled concentration, but with a soluble one equilibration is slow because of the rapid diffusion of molecules. Thus the "head of pressure" in the alveoli remains low, and so does the arterial tension.

The ultimate mechanism by which the anaesthetics produce their effect on the cells of the central nervous system is not known, as testified by the many theories on their action. We do know, however, that the brain is progressively affected by an anaesthetic in relation to its developmental structure. The "highest" areas are the first to lose their function, with the production of unconsciousness. At this point the sub-conscious mind, released from higher control, may give rise to unconscious struggling, shouting, and breath holding. This level of cerebral activity is next abolished, continuance of the anaesthetic leading to suppression of the reflex response of the patient to stimuli.

This loss of reflex activity is itself a graduated process. At first co-ordinated reflex movements are abolished; then muscle contraction in response to, first, stimulation of comparatively insensitive structures, and secondly, stimulation of sensitive areas of the body. For example, at a certain light level of anaesthesia incision of the skin of the abdominal wall will evoke no corresponding tightening of the abdominal muscles, but handling of the peritoneum at such a level would result in their immediate contraction. It is worth noting here that such a reflex response to stimulus under comparatively light anaesthesia may show itself in the less obviously related form of *laryngeal spasm* of varying degree, as well as disturbances in the rate and rhythm of respiration.

Types of Anaesthetic

Anaesthetics have two functions to perform: first the production of unconsciousness and consequent insensibility to pain; and secondly, the production of a motionless, flaccid field in which the surgeon can work to his, and therefore the patient's, best advantage. However, all anaesthetic drugs are poisons. Remember that in achieving a state of anaesthesia you intend to poison someone, but not kill them — so give as little as possible.

In most operations performed outside the abdominal cavity (and such extra-abdominal procedures form the bulk of surgical practice), the desired flaccidity may be maintained by a comparatively light level of anaesthesia. Such levels of anaesthesia do little harm to a patient and an untroubled post-operative period may be expected. In abdominal operations anaesthesia must either be maintained at a much deeper plane or, in modern practice with a skilled anaesthetist, the necessary abdominal relaxation is produced by a different agent — a muscle relaxant, or less commonly the use of a spinal or local block — using the general anaesthetic solely for the production of unconsciousness. This combination of drugs and methods avoids the use of large doses of toxic agents, with their inevitable complications and sequelae for the patient.

Thus, there are from the administrator's viewpoint three types of anaesthetic:

(i) *Light anaesthesia*, without profound muscular flaccidity, for most operations outside the abdominal cavity.

(ii) *Deep anaesthesia*, producing profound muscular flaccidity, mainly for operations within the abdominal cavity.

(iii) Light anaesthesia producing unconsciousness only, with profound muscular flaccidity obtained by another agent.

The level of anaesthesia required for (i) and (iii) is identical, so that there are only two main types of general anaesthetic that the student requires to master in order to deal with all except the most formidable surgery. However, it is advisable for him to have a working knowledge of the other methods employed to provide profound muscular flaccidity, including the use of muscle relaxants (see p. 55).

CHAPTER 2

The Patient

The anaesthetist should examine each of his patients before operation, but unfortunately in hospital practice this is not always possible. Even though the house-surgeon performs his routine examination you should examine all candidates for major operations yourself, and at least read the notes of all others the night before their visit to the theatre.

It is advisable to separate your patients into two classes:
(1) Fit adults.
(2) The young, the old, and the ill.

The second group usually requires much less anaesthetic than the first, though children commonly need a surprisingly large dosage in comparison with their size. Among the fit adults are to be found a group of "anaesthetic resistant" patients who require a markedly greater amount of anaesthetic than the normal individual. This group includes males of heavy build and those accustomed to regular heavy drinking. Such patients may require modification of a "simple" technique if difficulties are to be avoided.

When examining the subject for the next day's surgery make a point of placing him in one of the above sections. You should make particularly certain that you have summed up:
(1) The extent of his surgical condition.
(2) The extent of any co-existent condition.
(3) The efficiency of his respiratory and circulatory systems.
Always, therefore, enquire for:
(1) Cough.
(2) Sputum.
(3) Dyspnoea on moderate exertion.
(4) Orthopnoea (any increase in the number of pillows at night?).
(5) Swelling of the ankles.
(6) History of anginal pain.

And examine for:
(1) Mechanical cardiac lesions.
(2) Cardiac arrhythmias.
Which are interesting and must put you on your guard, but of less practical significance than
(3) Crepitations at the lung bases.
(4) Oedema (ankle or sacral).
(5) Enlarged liver.
(6) Distension of jugular veins, indicating an increased venous pressure.
Which with positive answers to your questions (3), (4), (5) above suggest a failing heart.
(7) Raised blood pressure.
(8) Sugar and albumen in the urine.
(9) Anaemia,
as well as making a careful examination of the lungs and upper air passages. Examine the trachea in the neck and observe the accessibility of the arm veins. Attention should be paid also to the teeth, since loose ones may become foreign bodies in the airway. Serious sepsis of the gums should be treated — an essential before major surgery. It is also advisable to ask about previous anaesthetics, noting any ill effects which could be ascribed to a particular drug or technique. Jaundice after a previous halothane anaesthetic (see p. 50) will exclude the use of this drug. Thus a decision may be made at this preliminary examination on the drugs and methods you will use.

As anaesthetist, it is your responsibility to state whether a patient is fit for operation or not. In deciding this you must weigh the severity and urgency of the operation against the state of the patient's health, which usually comes to mean against the state of his cardiovascular system. It is the *efficiency* of the circulation that must be taken into consideration, not solely the physical signs presented. A patient who can perform his usual daily tasks without distress is fit for an operation. A patient who can climb a flight of stairs without marked dyspnoea is similarly suited for surgery. Many patients in late middle age present a slight degree of hypertension, and possibly report a swelling of their ankles at night (you exclude all the extra-cardiac causes). These people can be guaranteed to face up to all but the most serious procedures, although it is advisable to give them a few days' rest in bed beforehand.

Beware the patient with long-standing sepsis (bronchiectasis for example), for the myocardium may be damaged. This is also the case in chronic anaemia. Here, a pre-operative transfusion of whole blood will increase the haemoglobin, but may well overload the heart. Beware also the retired policeman or the athlete run to seed, for these patients are not nearly so healthy as suggested by their appearance. Examine especially carefully those complaining of increasing dyspnoea or orthopnoea. Remember, though, that these symptoms can be caused also by disease of the respiratory system. Emphysema, extensive fibrosis of the lung from any cause, and excessive sputum can present problems to try the most skilful.

Adopt no hard-and-fast rule, but judge each case on its merits; and if you are at all in doubt as to the presence or significance of any physical sign, then call upon the assistance of a physician. Remember always to ask about *drugs* the patient may be taking (p. 127), and his sensitivity to drugs of any sort.

Patients should never be starved, nor purged before operations not calling for previous emptying of the bowel. Normal feeding may be continued until the day of operation, when a fast of four hours is imposed upon the patient after a light meal. The patient should certainly spend an early night before his operation, though it is not necessary to keep uncomplicated cases in bed for any longer period.

The mental attitude of the patient requires as much consideration as his physical condition. Never think of him as "No. 12. Gastrectomy. Theatre C. 9.30," but as "Bill Smith, bus driver, five kids, very worried about surviving his operation". The sudden transition from home to the strange, bare, and disciplined atmosphere of a hospital is enough to disturb the most adaptable personality. When there is the threat of an imminent operation hanging over the patient as well, his mental unrest, however strongly concealed, must be considerable. If a visit from the anaesthetist can put his mind at rest, it will do more good than any amount of premedication.

Don't be over-hearty or over-solemn with patients. Be cheerful and let them know that hundreds of people pass through the same experience every week without disaster. Above all, appear perfectly confident, however dishonest this makes you feel.

Premedication

You will undoubtedly have to prescribe premedication at some time though you never enter an operating theatre from the day you qualify. With modern anaesthetic techniques premedication is probably less important than it used to be, but the standard procedure has become hallowed by tradition and has changed little during the last quarter century. Classically, the two functions that premedication is expected to perform are:

(1) Drying up the secretions to the respiratory tract glands (including the salivary glands).

(2) Depressing the activity of the patient's central nervous system in order to facilitate the forthcoming anaesthesia.

Drying the patient's secretions. This function is commonly performed with atropine or hyoscine (scopolamine).

(1) Atropine dries up the secretion of the bronchial glands by inhibiting the parasympathomimetic action of acetyl choline. By the same action it inhibits the secretion of the salivary glands, so that patients receiving atropine premedication invariably suffer from dryness of the mouth.

Atropine is a powerful drug, and apart from the desired drying-up effect exhibits several incidental actions of importance:

(2) The pulse rate is increased. Pre-operative atropine may therefore prevent cardiac arrhythmia mediated by the vagal nerves.

(3) The secretions of the gut are decreased, which is not only an aid in abdominal surgery but helps to prevent vomiting during and after the anæsthetic.

(4) The movements of the gut are inhibited.

(5) The secretion of sweat is prevented, loss of heat from the body being thereby diminished (see p. 83).

(6) The pupil is dilated.

(7) Atropine causes a *stimulation* of the motor centres of the brain.

Hyoscine produces the same peripheral effect as atropine, the important difference between the two drugs being their action on the central nervous system. Hyoscine is a cerebral depressant which also causes a measure of amnesia, and indeed is frequently used for the control of maniacal excitement. Thus the use of hyoscine instead of atropine for premedication provides the two effects sought by the anaesthetist with a single drug. Also, many believe that hyoscine is a better drying agent than atropine, but the effect on the heart is less marked.

It is obvious that if non-irritating anaesthetic agents are used, which is common nowadays (e.g., the thiopentone, muscle relaxant, nitrous oxide — oxygen sequence), the need of drying up secretions is lessened. But when ether is administered — as it may well be in primitive surroundings — you will save embarrassment for yourself and danger to your patient by prescribing an antisialagogue. Equally, you will be advised to premedicate your patient with atropine or hyoscine to avoid cardiac arrhythmias. Thus the original drugs are still recommended, but, as so often the case in medicine, for a different reason.

Depressing the activity of the central nervous system. This is usually achieved by a dose of morphine administered with either atropine or hyoscine, which has the effect of:

(1) Depressing the higher centres of the brain, producing an inclination to sleep and an uncaring attitude towards the approaching operation.

(2) Relieving any pain the patient might be suffering, thus lowering his B.M.R., to the advantage of the anaesthetist.

(3) Depressing the respiratory centre;
    depressing the cough centre;
    stimulating the vomiting centre — all three disadvantageous during and after the administration.

(4) Slowing the pulse;
    constricting the pupil by stimulation of the third nerve nucleus — both these actions are antagonized by atropine or hyoscine.

Papaveretum (Omnopon) is often used in place of morphine, in the belief that it gives rise to less post-operative vomiting than the pure alkaloid. Omnopon consists of 50 per cent morphine and 50 per cent of the mixed alkaloids of opium. The dose is therefore twice the corresponding dose of morphine.

In those intolerant of morphine and those who are known to vomit severely after operation, morphine may be replaced by pethidine or one of the phenothiazine type of drugs (i.e., chlorpromazine, promezathine, etc. See p. 15).

Premedication producing sleep is usually referred to as *basal narcosis*, which is discussed in Chap. 5. We should, however, consider in this section the *oral barbiturates*, such as pentobarbitone (Nembutal), quinalbarbitone (Seconal), and amylobarbitone (Amytal).

These drugs are barbiturates of the short-acting class (see Chap. 5), their action beginning about half an hour from the moment of swallowing and persisting for some two hours longer. The drugs should produce complete unconsciousness, or at least an extreme drowsiness which will be associated with amnesia, but they have no analgesic properties. Occasionally, therefore, barbiturates produce excitement and uncontrollable restlessness — the response of the body, when no longer under voluntary control, to any form of stimulation (often no more than unexpected noises, lights, or movements just sufficient to disturb sleep). This is often seen when the effect of the drug is beginning to wear off, which is especially unfortunate if occurring during an operation being performed under local analgesia.

Recently, barbiturates and most of the phenothiazine drugs have been accused of having an "antanalgesic effect", making a person more sensitive to pain rather than less. They should not be withheld on this account.

Another disadvantage is the uncertainty of absorption from the stomach, with its associated difficulty in determining an effective dose. Although thiopentone is not precluded in the subsequent administration, it must be used with caution, since the accumulative effect of two barbiturates may cause severe depression, particularly of the respiratory centre.

Barbiturates have been recommended to accompany extensive local analgesia. Certainly they provide a restful state of mind, and by depressing the cortex protect the patient from possible toxic effects. But they also depress the heart.

Choice and Dosage of Premedication

The character of the premedication should be dictated by the type of anaesthesia which it is intended shall follow. If the patient is to inhale the agents by his own respiratory efforts, light premedication which does not depress respiration is indicated. On the other hand, this is immaterial if respiration is to be depressed deliberately (for example, with muscle relaxants), for it then becomes necessary for the patient's respiration to be assisted by the anaesthetist. Even so, heavy sedation is rarely advisable, since the effects may carry through into the postoperative period, delaying recovery from the anaesthetic and possibly endangering the patient's life. Inadvertent respiratory depression caused by the morphine group of drugs can be counteracted by naloxone (Narcan) or nalorphan (Lethidrone) in a dose of 10–20 mg. But if sedation without depression is wanted, then phenothiazine drugs like phenergan are useful.

Whatever the defects of morphine may be, it is unquestionably the drug of choice when the patient is in pain.

In deciding the type and dosage of your premedication, make use of the classification:

(1) Fit adults.
(2) The young, the old, and the ill.

(1) **Fit adults** (puberty to late middle-age — roughly 13 – 60). A well established and satisfactory premedication is:

morphine 15 mg
atropine 0·6 mg

or

Omnopon 15 mg
scopolamine 0·3 mg

(2) **The old** (over 65). With increasing years a more placid outlook on life may be expected, though unhappily often accompanied by a less efficient respiratory function, which is difficult to assess clinically. Heavy sedation is not only unnecessary, but may be dangerous.

A satisfactory injection is:

morphine 10 mg
atropine 0·6 mg

Patients past 80 are best prescribed atropine 0·6 mg.

(3) **The ill.** The ill, or shocked, may be treated like the old. It should never be necessary to exceed:

morphine 10 mg
atropine 0·6 mg,

but you must use your common sense about dosage. More often than not, desperately ill patients are best anaesthetized after premedication with atropine 0·6 mg alone. If you are ever in doubt over the correct premedication for an ill person, omit the morphine.

(4) **The young.** Morphine may be given safely by weight (mg 0·25/kg body weight), but the risk of a delayed recovery, especially where an early return to normal feeding is desired, may preclude its use. On the whole, it is best not to administer morphine below the age of 5 years. Atropine, on the other hand, is well tolerated by all ages.

If necessary, opium injection (paediatric), which contains the equivalent of 5 mg morphine/ml may be useful. The dose is calculated on the basis of 0·1 ml per year, conveniently but rather inaccurately, so great care is needed in measurement.

Phenothiazine Drugs

Recent years have seen the introduction of numerous "tranquillizers". They probably act on the reticular system of the brain, and may be expected to cause euphoria without respiratory depression, some protection of the body against shock, and some drying of secretions. Some have also an anti-adrenergic effect, counteracting the action of adrenaline by sympathetic blockade and causing vasodilatation with a fall in blood pressure. Chlorpromazine (Largactil), promezathine (Phenergan), and promazine (Sparine) are the most commonly used members of this group, and have antiemetic and antihistaminic properties as well. Of the two, promezathine is more predictable in its effects, and less likely to cause incidental hypotension and tachycardia — which is important, as the actions of both are prolonged and irreversible. Either drug is given in a dose of 50 mg intramuscularly one hour pre-operatively or by mouth two hours pre-operatively, and is often combined with pethidine. When non-irritant anaesthetic agents are employed, the antisialogogic effect of these drugs is adequate, but there is no protective action on the heart.

In some instances the hypotension caused is invoked deliberately to reduce operative bleeding. Such patients may look frighteningly pale and ill. This state of affairs is not for the inexpert. On the other hand, certain drugs which fall into this category have an almost specific anti-emetic effect, which may demand their use in the prevention or treatment of postoperative vomiting. Those popular for this purpose are perphenazine (Fentazin) 2·5–5·0 mg metoclopramide (Maxalon) 5·0–10 mg or prochloperazine (Stemetil) 12·5 mg.

Neuroleptics

Neuroleptic anaesthesia is receiving increasing attention, so some knowledge is necessary of the drugs used. From our describing these anaesthetics under premedication, you will appreciate that one state should run smoothly into the other.

Droperidol (Droleptan) is the usual basic drug for neuroleptic anaesthesia, but by itself tends to cause profound psychological depression. It is therefore combined with other drugs, sometimes a barbiturate, or fentanyl (Sublimaze). In choosing a mixture, remember that the effects of droperidol last for several hours but of fentanyl no more than thirty minutes. Extrapyramidal stimulation may be an undesirable consequence, but this can usually be controlled with diazepam (Valium). No matter what advantage may be claimed (and there are many, including a stable blood pressure) we warn strongly that these drugs are not for the beginner. Injudicious use can cause grave psychiatric disturbances.

Administration of Premedication

If premedication is to have any value at all, its timing is important. Subcutaneous atropine and hysocine begin to act after some 30 minutes and become fully effective within the next fifteen. Morphine acts rather more slowly, but the effects of both drugs may be expected to last for about 4 hours. Premedication should thus be given at least one hour before the patient is due to arrive in the anaesthetic room.

(1) **If premedication has not been given** in the ward it may be given intravenously in the anaesthetic room. By then the value of the sedative component will have been lost, and it may therefore be omitted.

(2) **Premedication given too late.** If the injection is obviously doomed to be administered too late, then the sister should withhold the drug for the anaesthetist to inject intravenously as above. If the drugs have unfortunately already been administered, the anaesthetic may be started, but a careful watch must be kept for the development of respiratory depression soon after induction.

(3) **Premedication given too early.** Nothing need be done for delays up to three hours. Thereafter atropine may be repeated, intravenously if more convenient, when a vagal-blocking effect is particularly desired.

Children

Psychologically there is much to be said for allowing the patient to become unconscious in his cot, often without knowledge that the operation is to take place.

There is a wide choice of premedication for children, but it is now customary to avoid needle pricks whenever possible. Trimeprazine tartrate (Vallergan), as a palatable syrup (6 mg/ml) given 1½ hours pre-operatively, is as useful as any. It is related to chlorpromazine and promezathine, and the dose is 3–4 mg/kg.

Barbiturates require two hours to become fully effective. It is advisable to prick the ends of capsules with a needle to facilitate absorption. Because of the bitter flavour, they should be restricted to children who can reasonably be expected to swallow them whole, but are no longer popular. If the child is in pain, morphine or pethidine should be given intramuscularly in amounts scaled down from the adult dose.

Atropine may be given half an hour before the induction is due to begin, the child by that time usually being asleep or drowsy enough not to recall the injection. It may be given orally with the sedative.

A convenient scheme of dosage for small children is:

0–6/12	atropine 0·3 mg	
6/12–2	atropine 0·4 mg	
2+	atropine 0·6 mg	+ sedation.

The patient must be moved gently from bed to the anaesthetic room, and in silence.

A sound sleep must be provided for the patient the night before his operation. Children usually sleep well, but adults should always be prescribed a mild sleeping draught. Butobarbitone (Soneryl) mg 200 is most satisfactory, although any drug to which the patient is accustomed, or is currently popular in the hospital, will suffice. If you want to avoid barbiturates, use nitrazepam (Mogadon) 5 mg.

But premedication is no longer thought to be absolutely essential, and in an emergency may be omitted altogether.

CHAPTER 3

The Airway

The first rule of anaesthesia is: *Keep a clear airway*. This is one of the "rules" of medicine of real and constant importance. It applies equally forcibly to cases when the general anaesthetic is *not* being administered through the lungs, and to patients who have left the table but not yet returned to full consciousness. It is applicable also to patients who are unconscious from any reason whatsoever.

If the airway becomes obstructed, not only is there danger of killing the patient but he becomes exhausted with his increased respiratory efforts. The signs of anaesthesia become unintelligible, partly due to oxygen lack and partly due to failure to eliminate carbon dioxide. And, if an inhalational anaesthetic is being employed, an insufficient amount of the agent finds its way into the lungs.

What is the "Airway"?

The airway extends from the bottom of the anaesthetist's oxygen cylinder to the endothelial walls of the capillaries surrounding the alveoli of the lung. There is therefore plenty of opportunity for obstruction to occur and much care is required in its avoidance.

Obstruction to the airway may be either partial (to any degree) or complete. It usually occurs suddenly, and demands prompt recognition, location, and relief.

The signs of obstruction are

(1) Diminution or absence of respiration, as shown by the reservoir bag. Often, the movements of the bag bear no relationship to the heaving efforts of the patient's chest or abdomen.

(2) Straining at inspiration, with indrawing of the soft tissues in the suprasternal notch and intercostal spaces.

(3) Use of the accessory muscles of inspiration (including the dilators of the external nares) if the patient is not deeply anaesthetized.

(4) "Tracheal tug" — a pulling down of the trachea and larynx with each attempted inspiration. This is not an invariable sign, and is discussed more fully below.

(5) A snoring or crowing noise.

(6) The possible supravention of cyanosis and the signs of hypoxia.

(7) Although noisy breathing means some degree of obstruction, complete obstruction is silent.

The most common cause of obstruction to the airway is the tongue falling back to meet the posterior pharyngeal wall; the second most frequent is laryngeal spasm. These and the other conditions causing obstruction will now be discussed, in their approximate order of frequency.

(1) Tongue falling back

This accident may occur at any time during the patient's period of unconsciousness, and must be particularly guarded against:

During induction.

When the patient is on the trolley in the recovery room or awaiting return to the ward.

After he has been replaced in bed.

The cause of the obstruction is usually revealed by the signs enumerated above being accompanied by a deep-toned snoring noise, but whatever you suspect to be the cause of your patient's distress always apply the treatment for this particular condition first — pull the jaw forward. That is, with the patient lying on his back you draw the point of the jaw towards the ceiling. This may be performed simply by two fingers under the symphysis mentis, although it may sometimes be easier to press forward the angles of the jaw with the thumbs. From this advice it is easily appreciable that the successful avoidance of this condition lies in conscientiously maintaining the point of the jaw forward during the entire administration. Indeed, the conventional grip for an anaesthetic mask includes the application of the second and third fingers to the point of the jaw, with the little finger hooked round the angle of the mandible if necessary.

It is surprising how often the simple action of drawing the jaw forward — and so, you will understand, pulling forward the tongue by its muscular attachments to the mandible — is successful in preventing what appears to be impending disaster. You may one day find yourself hurriedly called to the recovery room or ward to discover your last patient deeply cyanosed and under the energetic care of three nurses, the trio performing artificial respiration and administering oxygen with no effect. The only manoeuvre usually required is a stiff tug on the chin.

When your patient leaves the theatre always be certain that the nurse is effectively supporting the chin, and never release your own supporting fingers until you have delivered the patient to hers. These precautions may read as over-elaborate details, but each is highly important. Everyone in the theatre is busy at the end of an operation, the anaesthetist particularly, so that it is worth adopting the invariable habit of devoting one hand to supporting the patient's chin despite the occurrence of other pressing employment for both. Just as gravity allows the tongue to fall back and obstruct the patient who is lying on his back, so in the semi-prone or "tonsil" position it may be invoked to prevent this accident occurring. There is much to be said for the use of this position for any patient who has not yet recovered from his anaesthetic.

The artificial airway is designed to keep the tongue away from the posterior pharyngeal wall and the soft palate separated from the tongue. It may be manufactured in metal, plastic, or black rubber. These airways, well lubricated, are inserted upside down and turned to their normal position inside the mouth. It must be emphasized that the insertion of such pieces of apparatus does not release the anaesthetist or nurse from the obligation of supporting the jaw. Although in many cases a perfectly clear passage may be established after the insertion of an artificial airway, the patient very often remains partly obstructed until the mandible is pulled forward.

Occasionally the teeth are clenched so firmly that the insertion of an airway becomes impossible, a contingency likely to arise during induction, and at the end of a light anaesthetic. In such a case pass through the nares a length of cut Magill tube (No. 7 or 8 for an adult), advancing the tube as far as the hypopharynx. As soon as the tube passes the dorsum of the tongue, free breath sounds will be heard. Do not omit first to grease the tube, to take great care in its passage through the nose, and to fasten through its exposed end a safety-pin. The passage of a full-length Magill tube into the larynx will, of course, incidentally remove the threat of obstruction from the tongue, a patient once intubated requiring no support to the mandible.

But beware. The passage of tubes through the nose, though convenient on occasion, can easily cause a furious haemorrhage.

Ideally all patients should return to the ward via a recovery room, which must be next to the theatres. This avoids a dangerous journey through corridors and lifts when it is almost impossible to exercise proper supervision of the patient. Further, it ensures that the patient regains consciousness in the presence of specially trained personnel, with essential resuscitation and monitoring equipment to hand, and medical staff who know about the patient immediately available.

(2) Laryngeal spasm

This condition is particularly likely to arise during induction, though it may occur at any time during the administration or the recovery period. It can be either partial or complete. The diagnosis of partial laryngeal spasm is to be made from the signs of obstruction plus a characteristic high-pitched crowing from the larynx itself, which if lightly touched gives the sensation of handling a purring cat. The spasm, whether partial or complete, usually follows:

(i) *Irritation of the larynx by*:
(a) Too rapid increase in anaesthetic vapour, particularly the irritating vapour of ether.
(b) Blood, mucus, vomit.
(c) Foreign body, such as an airway or an endotracheal intubation attempted under too light anaesthesia.
(d) Direct irritation by the surgeon if for any reason the patient is not intubated.

(ii) *Reflex irritation of the larynx*.
The surgeon's manipulations in any part of the body may give rise to a reflex partial (or occasionally complete) laryngeal spasm if the level of anaesthesia is not sufficiently deep. Note that the depth of the anaesthesia is relative to the part handled, and that a plane of narcosis deep enough to avoid spasm from incision of the skin will allow pronounced spasm to follow such manoeuvres as handling of the testis, the peritoneum, or the under surface of the diaphragm, or dilating the cervix or anus.

(iii) *Hypoxia*.
Hypoxic muscle goes into spasm, and the adductors of the

vocal cords are no exception. Hence the "vicious circle"—spasm of the larynx produces oxygen lack, which in turn increases the laryngeal spasm to augment the hypoxia. This circle has obviously to be broken swiftly, by adopting the treatment outlined below.

(iv) *Use of intravenous barbiturates.*

The intravenous barbiturates, particularly thiopentone (which is the commonest in use today), can predispose to spasm of the larynx. This may be due to their anaesthetizing the sympathetic nervous system to a greater extent than the parasympathetic system. Whatever the mechanism, patients who have been induced with thiopentone sometimes exhibit spasm when the induction is continued with inhalation anaesthesia administered in too high a concentration, for which the so-called non-irritant vapours may not be blameless. Whether the spasm is direct or reflex, the effect of thiopentone in facilitating its occurrence may remain for a considerable time. This danger has probably been overstressed in the past but must be borne in mind, especially with sufferers from asthma, whose respiratory tract is unduly sensitive and will often respond vigorously to any form of mechanical irritation—laryngoscopy, intubation, etc.

It is worth remembering that the insertion of a pharyngeal airway immediately after induction with thiopentone may give rise to troublesome spasm, and that endotracheal tubes should never be passed under thiopentone alone. Also note—a dose of thiopentone may not only initiate laryngeal spasm, but will also depress respiration to an extent that completely obscures the picture of obstruction and prevents the performance of respiratory efforts. Indeed, this respiratory depression, invariable after all but the smallest doses of thiopentone, may produce a dangerous failure to make respiratory efforts whatever the cause of the obstruction. Remember, then, when using thiopentone—keep a clear airway.

Treatment of Laryngeal Spasm

Partial spasm.

If associated with the increase in anaesthetic vapour during induction, decrease the amount of vapour and repeat the induction. Sometimes a breath of fresh air will relieve the condition.

If associated with surgical interference, cautiously increase the depth of anaesthesia. Spasm may persist into deep anaesthesia, in which case, if you feel really confident of success, the passage of an endotracheal tube may be attempted.

In both cases see that the patient is receiving enough oxygen by increasing the percentage of oxygen in the mixture.

In both cases be sure to hold the jaw well forward in spite of your preoccupation with the larynx.

Complete Spasm.

This alarming condition is treated in the same way whenever it occurs.

   (i) Place one finger on the pulse; pull the jaw well forward. The airway as far down as the closed cords must be perfectly clear in order to allow the smallest inspiratory effort to be rewarded with a breath.

  (ii) Apply oxygen under moderate pressure. In this way, some oxygen will reach the lungs as soon as the cords begin to open.

 (iii) Stop all other interference with the patient.

With persistent spasm the pulse will rise and the patient become cyanosed. Be certain that the above conditions are strictly fulfilled, and they will in most cases be followed by the start of respiration and subsequent oxygenation of the patient. Attempts at intubation are more likely to aggravate than relieve the condition, and even if forcible efforts with a stiff catheter are made failure is almost certain. In complete spasm not only are the cords adducted but they are hidden by the aryepiglottic folds, which unite in the midline. The administration of a muscle relaxant will relax the spasm and permit intubation, and in skilled hands this is the correct treatment. For the less skilled, "masterly inactivity" as indicated above is preferable, in the knowledge that while there is spasm there is muscle tone and the patient must therefore still be alive. Spasm always relaxes before death.

Anoxia and carbon-dioxide retention will be severe, and can be particularly dangerous to a patient with a diseased heart. Remember that you can always ask the surgeon to perform an immediate tracheostomy if you feel the situation has gone beyond your control. Spasm cannot occur after intubation since the cords are held apart by the tube.

(3) Obstruction due to the patient's disease

Upper respiratory tract. When surgical anaesthesia has been established, a patient tends to breathe through his nose. At this level of anaesthesia trismus is not uncommon, so that inadequate nares become a troublesome condition.

Treatment: Insert an airway as soon as possible.

Englarged tonsils, adenoids, and so on all belong to this group.

Lower respiratory tract. You will probably be warned of the presence of such obstructions as the thyroid, an aneurism, etc., and if possible carefully pass a stiff Magill tube past the lesion. You should also know of pre-existent pulmonary fibrosis, bronchitis, and emphysema. Treat these, as all the conditions mentioned in the paragraph, with an excess of oxygen to allow no possibility of anoxia, but remember there is no substitute for effective ventilation.

(4) Obstruction due to substances entering the respiratory tract

The causes of this variety of obstruction are:

> sputum
> blood
> vomit
> foreign bodies,

which may enter either the upper or lower respiratory tract with equal effect.

(i) *Sputum* may be troublesome in any patient who is a heavy smoker or sufferers from the British complaint of bronchitis, but is most pronounced in those with bronchiectasis, whether they are undergoing lobectomy or any other operation. The danger of a large amount of sputum in the lower respiratory tract lies not only in the mechanical obstruction but in its spreading infection to uncontaminated parts of the lung. Mucus is as likely to cause obstruction as purulent sputum.

The recognition of sputum in the trachea and bronchi depends on distinguishing the rattle of the fluid with the respiratory movements. This sound is amplified by the breathing tubes of the apparatus, to which an ear may be applied in suspected cases. When the respiration is shallow, a small amount of sputum will not be so revealed, and its possible occurrence must be borne in mind in the event of obvious obstruction.

The application of a stethoscope to the chest, when practicable, will reveal any doubtful cases. It is especially valuable in small children, where a diaphragm stethoscope may be strapped to the chest preoperatively and left in position, or even better, an oesophageal stethoscope inserted. Ideally, patients should not undergo operation until their sputum has been reduced to an absolute minimum by vigorous preoperative treatment—postural drainage, breathing exercises, etc.

(ii) *Blood* may enter the trachea and bronchi from the lung or the upper respiratory tract, and its presence may be detected in the same way as above. Should there be a quantity of blood in the upper air passages the possibility of its descending past an insensitive larynx must be remembered. E.N.T. surgery is rich in such opportunities, and if there is any bleeding from the upper respiratory tract during or after an E.N.T. operation it must be made certain there is no chance of blood entering the trachea. The problem during operation has been largely solved by the introduction of endotracheal anaesthesia, but when the tube is removed at the end of the procedure see that the patient's head is depressed below his shoulders and/or he is light enough to possess an effective cough reflex.

(iii) The presence of *vomit* is to be feared on any occasion when emesis occurs while consciousness is lost, inhalation of the material occurring from the pharynx. Fortunately, the cough reflex is obtunded at a lower level of anaesthesia than the vomiting reflex, but obstruction is still possible—particularly in a shocked and feeble patient.

To avoid this accident:

(*a*) Make perfectly certain no food whatsoever has been taken during the four hours before operation, whatever the form of general anaesthesia contemplated and however trivial the operation. "Food" includes anything taken by mouth except small quantities of plain water. Particularly beware of milk, which is unique in solidifying instead of liquefying after ingestion, and may cause great difficulty in its removal when vomited into the pharynx. Suspect all children, who must be separated from temptation in the form of bars of chocolate and so forth in their hospital locker. And suspect all mothers, who must be made to understand in the out-patient department that if little Willie has been slipped a surreptitious currant bun, then only open confession can save his life. Fear, or the accident which brings the patient to hospital, delays the emptying time of the stomach. Too rigid definition of a safe interval can be misleading.

(*b*) Don't take too long over your induction, which may leave your patient in the optimum level of anaesthesia for vomiting for a dangerously long period. Don't persist in passing airways and tubes under too light anaesthesia. And remember — an adult will cough in response to such inopportune stimulation, but a child will probably vomit.

(c) Watch that the patient does not become too light during the operation, particularly when anaesthetizing children, whose first marked sign of lightening anaesthesia is often a brisk emesis.

(d) Watch for the signs of impending vomiting:
salivation, which may be obscured by the premedication,
swallowing, most frequently seen,
pallor, possibly, and
preliminary *retching*.

(e) If vomiting occurs:
Keep the airway as clear as possible by pulling forward the jaw.
Turn the patient's head to one side, or better still, the patient.
Raise the patient's feet.
If inhalation has not occurred, rapidly clear away the vomit from the mouth and, if induction is taking place, continue deepening the anaesthetic. In any event keep the patient's head down. Don't worry about the vomit on the pillow. It may be messy, but it's not dangerous — it's the vomit still inside which is important.

(f) Anticipated vomiting, when proper precautions have been taken, is not nearly so dangerous as the unexpected. Assume that all children and maternity cases will vomit and be prepared accordingly.

(g) Do not forget that patients may regurgitate silently, especially after muscle relaxants. This can occur without warning, usually during induction. It must always be remembered as a risk during labour, where there is a hiatus hernia, and in cases of intestinal or oesophageal obstruction. The quantity of fluid may be small in the labouring mother owing to restricted intake, but the highly acid stomach contents produce an alarming effect on the lungs (see p. 105).

(iv) *Foreign bodies* dropping past an insensitive larynx may include teeth, tonsils, unconnected endotracheal tubes, and so forth.

All these agents may not only give rise to obstruction, but, if not efficiently removed, a subsequent bronchopneumonia or lung abscess.

Treatment. When any of the above materials are discovered to be in the bronchial tree there must be removed. The first step is to raise the patient's feet. Next, aspirate the material. Often, it is best to pass an endotracheal tube first, deepening the anaesthesia if necessary and practicable. Then pass through the tube a rubber catheter attached to a suction apparatus, or to a bladder syringe if no apparatus is available. Common sense must be used in every case. A lightly anaesthetized patient, for example, will cough up a little sputum at the end of the operation, and it is not necessary to disturb him to the extent already outlined. Conversely, a large amount of material suddenly entering the bronchial tree, particularly if it is solid rather than liquid, or any material not undergoing successful removal, demands prompt suction through a bronchoscope.

Note. Except in great emergency, suction should never be applied to the endotracheal tube itself owing to the risk of applying a dangerously high negative pressure to the lungs.

This is, perhaps, the best point to consider the infrequent but serious condition of *pulmonary oedema*. This emergency can occur with surprising suddenness on the table, and may be due to:

(*a*) Usually, acute heart failure, possibly the result of over-loading the circulation with intravenous fluids, or pressure alterations in any chamber of the heart or the carotid sinus.

(*b*) Prolonged respiratory obstruction.

Excess fluid must be aspirated as often as necessary and oxygen given, preferably under pressure. In practice, this usually means intubating the patient and establishing intermittent positive pressure respiration. Aminophylline 250 mg should be given intravenously. As soon as possible, the patient should be raised into the sitting position (cf., any case of cardiac failure). Perform a phlebotomy of 200–300 ml, to reduce the load on the heart, when failure has been precipitated by over-transfusion. The intravenous injection of frusemide (Lasix) will quickly remove much unwanted fluid by promoting a vigorous diuresis, provided there is good renal function.

Pharyngeal Obstruction. Sputum, blood, vomit, and foreign bodies may give rise to dangerous obstruction *above* the larynx, an obstruction commonly associated with some degree of laryngeal spasm.

Treatment. Raise the patient's feet and rapidly remove any material in the mouth and pharynx, using your fingers and/or a suction apparatus if available; pull the jaw well forward; if there remains more material lower down the pharynx insert a laryngoscope and remove the offending matter with sucker, swab, or (in the case of foreign bodies) Magill forceps. Remember that if the patient is coughing it is unlikely any material will be inhaled, and if the patient is not coughing it is likely that material will be inhaled.

Remember also that the capacity of the bronchial tree is small, and that a foreign body (e.g., an inhaled piece of vomited apple) can cause complete obstruction by lodging at the larynx or in the trachea.

(5) Mechanical faults

Obstruction (let us for classification's sake give the condition a wide meaning) may occur from any of these faults in the apparatus:

(i) Oxygen cylinder run out.

(ii) Delivery tube kinked or leant upon by anaesthetist or surgeon.

(iii) Endotracheal tube —

(a) Kinked in pharynx or at teeth.

(b) Proximal end abutting against face mask, if also used.

(c) Bevel of distal end abutting against wall of trachea, especially when head is extended.

(d) Attached to twisted or compressed rubber adapting tube.

(e) Filled with blood clot or sputum (old or new) — this may apply also to an artificial airway.

Less commonly —

(iv) Reducing valve jammed

(v) flowmeter needle valve jammed

(vi) leak of gas flow, usually owing to failure to replace bottle after filling.

Note: If you are worried about your patient, and his condition is not improving in response to resuscitative efforts with your machine, then abandon the machine. Let him breathe the same air that you are breathing, but be sure he is doing so with equal lack of obstruction.

You must be careful not to confuse respiratory failure and obstruction. On this text let us consider:

What to do if the Patient Stops Breathing

This may be due to four cases:
(1) Obstruction.
(2) Too deep — respiratory failure.
(3) Too light — breath holding.
(4) The effect of relaxants.
The anaesthetist will know if a relaxant has been given.
Examine for the first three causes in order.

(1) Obstruction
   (i) Arrest usually sudden.
  (ii) Inspiratory efforts usually being made.
 (iii) Cause of obstruction may be obvious.
Treatment. Look for cause and treat as above.

Note: Most cases are relieved by pulling the jaw forward.

(2) Too deep
   (i) The arrest is usually not sudden, but follows a period of decreasing respiratory volume.
  (ii) The signs of deep anaesthesia are present (note the extreme muscle flaccidity, the dark blood, and if necessary confirm by looking at the size of the pupils).
 (iii) A relatively large amount of anaesthetic has been given.

Treatment.
   (i) Be sure the airway is clear.
  (ii) Cut off the anaesthetic.
 (iii) Perform artificial respiration until normal breathing is established.
 (iv) Administer oxygen if available.

(3) Too light
The arrest is sudden, though it may be preceded by respiratory irregularities, and is usually obviously related to surgical stimulus. The other signs of light anaesthesia are present. This cause is frequently operable in induction in · response to too rapid increase in vapour strength.
Treatment. Remove the anaesthetic vapour and allow the patient to breathe air or oxygen until regular respiration begins again. Then gently reintroduce the anaesthetic vapour and deepen the narcosis. Squeezing the bag may hasten this process.

Let us also discuss

Cyanosis

First, understand this: Cyanosis is a condition in which there is a blue colouration of the skin and mucous membranes, and occurs when there is more than 5 g of reduced haemoglobin circulating in each 100 ml blood. Cyanosis is therefore not a condition relative to the degree of hypoxia. A person with only 5 g of haemoglobin per 100 ml blood (about "30 per cent") will die of anoxia but can never become cyanosed. A person with 20 g of haemoglobin per 100 ml blood (about "130 per cent") will become cyanosed though still possessing, in a fully oxygenated state, an amount of haemoglobin equal to the total of a normal person. So to the anaesthetist cyanosis is a warning that hypoxia is possibly occurring, but the absence of cyanosis does not mean that such hypoxia is not possible. Again use your common sense and take each case on its merits.

Cyanosis may be observed best in the lobes of the ears; then the lips (remember about lipstick in out-patients); the nails (always applicable to coloured patients); and, of course, best of all in the blood itself. Never ignore cyanosis. Always relieve it immediately. And remember that the condition may be cardiac in origin, so that the first step in treating a cyanosed patient is to place a finger on the pulse.

Note. If the patient becomes cyanosed during induction, check your gas and oxygen leads and cylinders. This must be done as a preliminary to any anaesthetic, but it does no harm to repeat the check.

Hypoxia

Oxygen lack may be due to:

Failure in supply of oxygen (including obstruction).

Failure in access of oxygen to the lungs (obstruction or respiratory disease).

Failure of the circulation taking oxygen to the tissues.

Failure of tissues to utilize oxygen.

Another cause for hypoxia has been recognized recently—*diffusion anoxia*[1] after nitrous oxide anaesthesia. The gas diffuses from the blood into the lungs in such quantity it displaces much of the alveolar air, leaving the patient an hypoxic mixture to breathe. This state of affairs may be aggravated by depressed

---

[1] Anoxia is total oxygen lack, hypoxia less than total. Diffusion anoxia is a technical term.

repiration and collapse of parts of the lungs. The treament is giving oxygen, which is recommended after all major surgery or when the patient is suffering from any respiratory or cardiac insufficiency.

The signs of hypoxia are:
(1) Slight degree of hypoxia.
    (i) Bounding pulse.
    (ii) Bleeding increased.
    (iii) Muscle spasm.
(2) Severe degree of hypoxia.
    (i) Failing pulse.
    (ii) Bleeding decreased.
    (iii) Usually cyanosis.

If there is hypoxia, there may well be carbon-dioxide retention at the same time. Look out, therefore, for sweating, deep breathing, and raised blood pressure in the early stages — and respiratory depression later.

Tracheal Tug

This condition, in which the trachea is pulled down with each inspiration, occurs:
(1) When there is an obstruction to inspiration.
(2) In serious respiratory depression (due to deep anaesthesia or other centrally acting drugs).
(3) When there is no obstruction to inspiration but the muscles are flaccid due to the action of a muscle relaxant. This is likely to be most obvious post-operatively, and is caused by a prolonged action of the relaxant. If this effect is not readily reversed by neostigmine (Prostigmin), then some abnormal response to the relaxant through electrolyte disturbance, metabolic acidosis, latent myasthenia gravis, or hypothermia, may be suspected.
Or
(4) A combination of the above.

Seek the cause and remove it if possible. When the depth of anaesthesia is at fault, lighter anaesthesia, or assisting respiration by squeezing the bag to coincide with inspiration, will decrease the jerky movement that is probably interfering with the surgeon.

CHAPTER 4

Signs of Anaesthesia

As noted in the first chapter, there are two functions required of a general anaesthetic. First, there is the production of narcosis and insensibility to pain, and secondly the provision of a motionless and unresisting field for the surgeon.

The depth of anaesthesia for this second requirement naturally varies with the operation. The drawing of a tooth or the incision of an abscess, for example, may be satisfactorily accomplished under extremely light anaesthesia. Operations within the abdominal cavity, however, require a deeper level of narcosis to abolish the tone of the abdominal muscles and prevent their reflex contraction in response to the surgeon's handling the sensitive peritoneum. Again, so is a varying level of anaesthesia needed to prevent reflex response to the operation on areas of the body of different sensitivity. In thoracotomy, for example, the lightest level of surgical anaesthesia is sufficient for the incision of the superficial structures, but interference with the periosteum of the ribs requires deeper narcosis to prevent the onset of reflex coughing.

Although the levels of anaesthesia have been stated by one forthright anaesthetist as "awake, asleep, dead," it is customary to divide the progress of the patient towards deep unconsciousness into certain stages and planes. The enumeration of the levels of narcosis was first made by Snow[1], but those listed here and usually referred to today were described by Guedel.

Stage 1. Stage of Analgesia
Pain dulled but consciousness retained.

[1] John Snow (1813–1858) was the first London professional anaesthetist. Of a fertile and logical mind, he achieved the first truly scientific approach to the subject. He is remembered particularly for his books on ether and chloroform, and for his administration of chloroform to Queen Victoria on the birth of Prince Leopold — an occasion quite obviously deciding in the current controversy that God had not, after all, constructed woman with the object of achieving painful parturition.

32

Stage 2. Stage of Excitement

Consciousness lost, but little change in pain perception. The abolition of higher controlling centres allows subconscious manifestations, and an over-reaction to all forms of stimulation (noise, bright lights, touch, pain), leading to breath holding, shouting, limb movement, and fighting.

Stage 3. Stage of Surgical Anaesthesia

Plane 1
Plane 2
Plane 3
Plane 4

Stage 4. Stage of Impending Overdose

Leading to failure of respiration followed by failure of the circulation.

These stages and planes are all correlated to physical signs. They were, however, originally described in relation to open ether anaesthesia without any premedication and cannot be strictly adapted to a modern anaesthetic administered by a different method and employing different drugs. The student may therefore find it easier to apply his physical signs to the following classification:

(1) **Inadequate Anaesthesia**

(2) **Surgical Anaesthesia**
    (i) Light
    (ii) Deep

(3) **Deep Anaesthesia**

The depth of unconsciousness is judged mainly from the respiration, additional information being obtained from the eyes. Much, too, can be learned from observing the response of the patient to stimulation. (Regardless of Guedel's stages and planes of anaesthesia, if the patient reacts to the surgeon's manipulations he is too light; if he does not, then at least he is sufficiently deep.) Note that deep general anaesthesia — whatever drugs are employed to achieve it — will have a bad effect on the patient. This will become obvious in the post-operative period, when the upset to normal metabolism delays full recovery. Deep anaesthesia should generally be practised only on fit, healthy patients undergoing short procedures.

The Respiration Under Anaesthesia

Note. Inspiration is performed by the action of the diaphragm and intercostal muscles. In the normal conscious patient diaphragmatic respiration predominates in the male and costal respiration in the female. Expiration is normally passive.

While respiration remains under conscious or subconscious control of the patient (i.e., in Guedel's 1st and 2nd stages) it may present any character from breath holding to tachypnoea, or may appear perfectly regular. The onset of automatic respiration, however, usually signals entry into the plane of surgical anaesthesia. These automatic respirations are completely regular, of a little faster rate and greater depth than the respirations of the conscious subject, and are, with a little experience, easily recognizable.

It is established that the patient has passed from the stage of inadequate anaesthesia to that of surgical anaesthesia by the onset of the characteristic automatic breathing; it remains to be decided whether the surgical anaesthesia is light or deep. If the patient's chest is moving, the intercostal muscles are working and the surgical anaesthesia is light. If the patient's chest is not moving and the respiration is being carried on entirely by the diaphragm, as shown by movement of the abdomen with each respiration, then the surgical anaesthesia is deep. These important signs must be looked for carefully. If the student is in doubt if the chest is moving or not he should lay a hand on the thoracic wall under the sterile towels.

Where the abdominal respiration begins to show a progressive decrease in volume, and perhaps takes on a jerky character and exhibits loss of regularity, then the stage of deep anaesthesia has been entered. Unless the anaesthesia is lightened respiration will cease.

From observation of the respiration alone the student may therefore form a pretty exact opinion of the depth of anaesthesia to which he has brought his patient. Additional information is obtained from the eyes, although pupillary signs are less reliable than respiratory ones.

The Pupil

(1) Position

The pupils may be observed moving or fixed in any position of squint until light surgical anaesthesia has been firmly established. They then take up a central position in the palpebral fissure, which they retain for the remainder of the anaesthesia.

To correlate the physical signs: if respiration is regular, the chest is moving, and the pupils are central, then light surgical anaesthesia has been firmly established. If the pupils are squinting and the respiration not automatic, then the anaesthesia is still inadequate for surgery.

(2) Size

An overdose of anaesthetic usually produces enlargement of the pupil owing to paralysis of the third nerve nucleus. The enlargement is not sudden, and is best noticed by comparing the size of the pupil at intervals of one or two minutes. If the respiration is abdominal in character and the pupil is large, then an overdose is being administered and respiration will shortly cease. It must be remembered, however, that there are three common causes of a dilated pupil in anaesthetic practice, all reasonably easy to distinguish:

(i) Overdose of anaesthetic.
(ii) Induction (due to subconscious fear, outpouring of adrenalin).
(iii) Premedication with atropine (usually seen where no morphine has been administered in addition, as in the case of young children).

In addition, two other causes, other signs of which will be obvious, may be encountered:

(iv) Severe hypoxia.
(v) Shock and haemorrhage.

(3) Reflexes

The eyelash. This is a useful guide for the anaesthetist. If one gently touches the eyelash of the conscious patient a reflex winking of the eye results. This reflex persists just as far as the onset of surgical anaesthesia. If the reflex is present, therefore, anaesthesia is inadequate for the surgeon. The reflex should be sought gently, as the semi-conscious patient may otherwise be precipitated into a state of excitement.

The conjunctiva and cornea. Although responding to stimulation until moderately deep anaesthesia, these reflexes should not be sought. The risk of damage to the eye is out of all proportion to their diagnostic value.

It is by careful observation of the above signs that the student can decide the depth of anaesthesia to which his patient is subjected, and he is well advised to check them several times during each administration.

Diagnosis of the Depth of Anaesthesia

The questions that the student most frequently has to ask himself in this respect are:

(1) Is the patient unconscious?
(2) Is he ready for the operation to begin?
(3) Is the anaesthetic becoming too deep?
(4) Is the anaesthetic becoming too light?

(1) Is the patient unconscious?

The exact moment that the patient loses consciousness is difficult to determine, particularly if the induction is performed slowly. The onset of true automatic breathing, however, indicates that the patient has entered the state of surgical anaesthesia, and is therefore certainly unconscious. If the patient makes purposeless movements or vague attempts to remove the mask, one may be consoled that consciousness has been lost. At the same time, it is advisable to remember that hearing is the last of the senses to disappear under anaesthesia, and one should avoid frightening the semi-conscious patient by talking to the nurse before narcosis is obviously established. The use of the intravenous barbiturates for the induction of anaesthesia has greatly modified the previously described progression from the stage of analgesia to that of excitement and then into the first plane of surgical anaesthesia, in that the patient is brought from the state of complete wakefulness to that of comparatively deep, though temporary, surgical anaesthesia in a matter of seconds (see p. 42).

(2) Is he ready for the operation to begin?

The answer to this depends entirely upon the operation to be performed. As already stated twice, from the anaesthetist's viewpoint operations may be divided into two classes:

(i) Those when the patient may be maintained lightly asleep to prevent the occurrence of interfering reflex movements.

(ii) When the patient must be deeply anaesthetized to prevent the occurrence of interfering reflex movements.

There is also subdivision (iii) when the patient may be lightly narcotized and the prevention of interfering reflex movements accomplished by another agent. The level of general anaesthesia required is the same as that called for by operation (i).

To return to our classification, then:

Light surgical anaesthesia suitable for (i) and (iii) is marked by:
(i) Respiration which is:
  (*a*) regular
  (*b*) thoracic.
(ii) Pupils which are:
  (*a*) fixed
  (*b*) central
  (*c*) usually not dilated.
(iii) Reflexes:
  (*a*) eyelash reflex absent.

Watch the patient carefully as the first incision is made. If he is lightly anaesthetized, even to a depth satisfactory for the operation, the respiration will quicken or perhaps falter momentarily at this initial stimulus, while the pulse rate will probably show a slight rise. If the patient's respiration suddenly ceases or becomes highly irregular, of if there is reflex movement or laryngeal spasm (see p. 21), then the anaesthesia is too light and must be deepened for the tranquil continuance of the operation.

Deep surgical anaesthesia suitable for (ii) is marked by:
(i) Respiration which is:
  (*a*) regular
  (*b*) abdominal.
(ii) Pupils which are:
  (*a*) fixed
  (*b*) central
  (*c*) usually not dilated.
(iii) Reflexes: absent.

Watch the patient closely when the peritoneum is incised. Then you can see if the abdominal muscles remain slack under the surgeon's hands.

(3) Is the anaesthetic becoming too deep?

An overdose of anaesthetic is marked by:
(i) Respiration becoming irregular, shallow, or absent (see p. 29), other causes being excluded.
(ii) Pupils usually dilated.
(iii) Muscular tone absent, especially as shown by a flaccid abdominal wound.

The amount of anaesthetic already administered must obviously give you some rough guide to the probable depth of your patient's narcosis, but let it be merely a rough guide and nothing more. Patients vary surprisingly in the amount of anaesthetic they require to bring them to a particular level, and it is patently dangerous to judge the performance of an all-in wrestler, an old lady, and a new-born baby on the same scale. Never give more than is absolutely necessary for the particular operation. The anaesthesia is deep enough if the surgeon can carry out his duties unhindered by the patient.

(4) Is the anaesthetic becoming too light?

In an abdominal operation performed under general anaesthesia the first indication of the narcosis becoming too light is a tightening of the abdominal wall in response to the surgeon's stimulus, an eventuality he will lose no time in bringing to your notice. Note that the anaesthesia may remain satisfactory at a constant level, but the surgical stimulus may become suddenly increased and produce reflex response. For instance, all may go well during the manoeuvres of an abdominal operation, but at the final handling of the peritoneum for closure the level of anaesthesia will have to be increased to overcome the considerably augmented stimulus. It is in the anticipation of such movements, with a corresponding adjustment in the level of the narcosis, that a great part of the art of anaesthesia lies.

If, however, the peritoneum is not opened, indication that the anaesthesia is becoming too light is given by any of these signs:

(i) Respiratory rate increasing or becoming irregular.
(ii) Respiration ceasing suddenly.
(iii) Laryngeal spasm occurring.
(iv) The patient making a movement in response to stimulus. (It is advisable not to allow this sign to occur with an unsympathetic surgeon.)

At the same time the patient will have shown the signs of light surgical anaesthesia — the respiration will have been costal in type and the pupils possibly divergent. Remember that reflexes return at a lighter level of unconsciousness than that at which they disappear.

It must be clearly understood that all the above signs indicate the ability or failure to contract of a muscle or group of muscles. With deepening anaesthesia a progressive muscular depression takes place, and until the stage of respiratory arrest is reached the changing character of the respiration with the patient breathing *spontaneously* is the most valuable yardstick. But interference with this normal pattern can be effected by assisting, or more usually controlling, respiration by squeezing the bag of the anaesthetic machine. At first this must be done in time with the patient's respiration, but soon it will be possible for the anaesthetist to impose whatever rhythm he desires on the patient. This is achieved by "washing-out" the carbon dioxide and removing the normal respiratory stimulus (hyperventilation). Not only does this obscure the signs of anaesthesia, but may also provide some muscular relaxation by itself.

Similarly, but to a much greater extent, when muscles are paralysed by a muscle relaxant (or, indeed, an extensive local analgesic block) administered at the same time as a general anaesthetic, the guiding signs no longer exist. The anaesthetist now must rely entirely on his experience in deciding whether more or less anaesthetic drug is necessary for the patient (the clinical equivalent of "flying with the seat of the pants"). Occasionally slight lacrimation and a rise in pulse rate will give some indication that the level of anaesthesia is too light.

The anaesthetic may indeed become so light that the patient wakes up, yet is incapable of warning anyone of his predicament. Such nightmare incidents have occurred too often, causing the patient great mental if not physical anguish. Take care to avoid them.

CHAPTER 5

The Anaesthetic Drugs

We will consider the agents with which you must become familiar:

> nitrous oxide
> the intravenous barbiturates
> halothane
> trichlorethylene
> ether

and mention others of less importance to the student:

> the muscle relaxants
> hypotensive drugs
> cyclopropane
> chloroform
> methoxyflurane

as well as discussing an important gas in anaesthetic practice:

> carbon dioxide.

Nitrous Oxide

A gas heavier than air, compressed into cylinders as a liquid, and used mainly for dentistry, minor operations, and as a vehicle for stronger anaesthetic vapours.

Advantages

(i) Safety. The safest anaesthetic known, provided it is administered with an adequate supply of oxygen, with no specific effect on the respiratory or cardiovascular systems.

(ii) Non-flammable.

(iii) Non-irritant to the patient, and pleasant to inhale.

(iv) Very rapid in action and in elimination, therefore ideal when the patient wishes to go straight home.

(v) Post-operative sequelae, including vomiting, almost unknown.

Disadvantages

   (i) It is impossible to bring the patient to a plane lower than very light surgical anaesthesia with nitrous oxide alone, therefore its use is restricted.

 (ii) Anoxia must often be tolerated for a short time in order to provide anaesthesia solely with nitrous oxide.

(iii) Attempts to provide deep anaesthesia, and otherwise exceed the limitations of nitrous oxide anaesthesia, will lead to serious cerebral anoxia. The results of this are permanent if not lethal and must not even be considered.

(iv) Induction with nitrous oxide is unpleasant to some patients, probably more from the mask on the face than the gas itself.

Particular dangers

Bearing in mind the last paragraph, never administer nitrous oxide (mixed with either oxygen or air) for longer than 2–3 minutes without a reinforcing drug. Never use it alone on subjects with severe cardiac or pulmonary disease or anaemia, nor for young children.

Uses

(1) Alone, combined with oxygen, or more rarely nowadays, air. A possible combination for dentistry, minor operations such as the opening of an abscess or the setting of a Colles's fracture, and in midwifery. For the technique of nitrous oxide in obstetrics see p. 130.

(2) For induction of anaesthesia. In this case the administration of nitrous oxide is simpler than in the above circumstances, for the patient is already under the influence of premedication. Hold the mask above and away from the patient's face, allowing the gas to fall on to his nose and mouth. Administer pure gas at the rate of some eight litres a minute by the flow-meter, watch the patient's respiration and colour, and talk reassuringly and soothingly to him until you are certain consciousness is lost. When the respiration becomes regular apply the mask firmly to the face and simultaneously continue the induction with a more powerful drug (e.g., trichlorethylene or halothane), reduce the nitrous oxide to six litres a minute, and add oxygen at the rate of two litres a minute. Cyanosis is not a sign of nitrous oxide anaesthesia. It implies asphyxia and should be avoided at all costs.

(3) During maintenance of anaesthesia. As explained later

(p. 63), nitrous oxide is used in the production of deep anaesthesia as a vehicle for the carriage of a much stronger anaesthetic vapour to the patient. It must be understood that in such circumstances the gas is hardly acting as an anaesthetic at all. When, however, a light anaesthetic is desired, as for an orthopaedic or superficial operation, gas usually has a sufficient anaesthetic effect on the patient. Nitrous oxide may thus be administered to maintain an already established light narcosis, in the form of a 6:2 mixture with oxygen, or with the addition of small amounts of anaesthetic vapour, such as trichlorethylene or halothane.

Such light narcosis will be sufficient to keep a patient asleep, while conditions for major surgery are provided by the additional use of a muscle relaxant. As the patient will be paralysed, ventilation is essential. But be warned again: too light a narcosis will let the patient become unpleasantly aware of his predicament.

(4) Nitrous oxide is available as pre-mixed nitrous-oxide–oxygen in equal concentrations. This is achieved by invoking some interesting but complicated physico-chemical properties, so that, unless the cylinder is cooled below freezing point, the emerging mixture is always constant. It is sufficient for analgesia, and is thus of value in obstetrics (see p. 130). It is used increasingly by ambulance men in extracting the injured from crashed vehicles, and for transporting patients in pain. It may also be used as a vehicle for a stronger anaesthetic vapour, especially in portable apparatus. Its main virtue is an assured, safe concentration of oxygen which cannot be varied.

The Intravenous Barbiturates

These are drugs of the ultra-short-acting group, used mainly for the pleasant induction of anaesthesia and for short anaesthesia in minor surgery.

Advantages
(i) Induction with thiopentone is by far the least unpleasant to the patient.
(ii) The drug is, naturally, non-irritant to the lungs and non-explosive.

Thiopentone is the commonest of the series in current use, but methohexitone enjoys some popularity because of rapid recovery — invaluable in a busy out-patient department.

(iii) A minimum of apparatus is required.
(iv) There are no unpleasant sequelae and vomiting is rare.
(v) Profound, though temporary, muscular relaxation may be rapidly achieved with a single dose.

Disadvantages

(i) Respiratory depression. This is marked with the barbiturates.
(ii) Hypotension. A fall in blood pressure is not unusual, and may be serious in cases of shock or where the cardiovascular system is diseased.
(iii) In common with other barbiturates, thiopentone is a good hypnotic, but a poor analgesic. Relatively large quantities are needed to produce true anaesthesia.
(iv) The recovery period is long in relation to the amount of thiopentone administered. Even after a minor procedure for which quite a small dose is given, drowsiness will ensue for an hour or so. But if followed by nitrous oxide, an even small dose will be adequate. The use of nitrous oxide for such minor surgery and dentistry in place of thiopentone has the advantage of allowing the patient to return home immediately.
(v) Difficulty in entering a vein. See hints on intravenous work on p. 85.
(vi) Laryngeal spasm. As already mentioned (p. 22) thiopentone renders the patient prone to laryngeal spasm which may prove dangerous if not correctly treated.
(vii) Major surgery under thiopentone alone should not be permitted.

Particular dangers

(i) "The danger with intravenous anaesthetics is that they are so fatally easy to give." Unlike the other general anaesthetics, thiopentone is not excreted by the body to any degree, recovery from a dose being dependent on the destruction of the drug by metabolic processes. A dose introduced into the circulation cannot be recovered, and an overdose once given cannot be detoxicated by the body it has poisoned. A little care and thought should preclude this action, though it must be remembered that "the young, old, and ill" require very much less of the drug than normal adult patients. Although age by itself is no contraindication to the use of thiopentone, the student is advised to proceed with great caution or even to avoid its use completely in patients at the extremes of age, and those enfeebled by illness. Whenever doubtful about the probable effects of the intravenous injection the procedure may be performed slowly, bearing in mind that the *normal* arm-brain circulation time is between ten and thirty seconds and watching the patient's respiration carefully for the effect of the drug. Remember that thiopentone, like other barbiturates, has a direct depressant effect on the heart. Thus a slow circulation time should warn of a poor cardiovascular system, and the need to avoid unnecessary added depression.

(ii) Thiopentone is a powerful respiratory depressant, the respiration ceasing in response to a moderate dose although the circulation continues without danger. To avoid trouble from this property of the drug bear in mind:

(a) A dose of thiopentone administered rapidly has a much more powerful transitory effect than an equal dose given slowly. This is because the rich blood supply to the brain carries such a high proportion of the dose to that organ, upon which it produces a profound effect before its subsequent redistribution through the other tissues. If the dose is given slowly the redistributive process will take place during the administration.

(b) The cumulative effect of thiopentone after other respiratory depressants, of which morphine is a common example. Thiopentone injected during the administration of another general anaesthetic may similarly produce respiratory failure in comparatively small dosage. The drug itself has a cumulative effect, smaller and smaller amounts requiring to be injected if the system of repeated doses is adopted. After the pre-operative administration of other short-acting barbiturates (e.g., quinalbarbitone) special care is needed.

(c) Always keep a clear airway after the injection of thiopentone, and administer artificial respiration if the natural breathing ceases. When administering this drug always be certain that you have a means of inflating the lungs available. Artificial respiration with oxygen or air is the most important action in treating such respiratory failure: a respiratory stimulant will not restart breathing and is no substitute for the inflation of the lungs.

(d) Bemegride (Megimide) will counteract depression caused by barbiturates. It is not a specific barbiturate antagonist, but is less likely to cause convulsions than the more usual analeptics — e.g., nikethamide (Coramine). The dose is up to 50 mg intravenously, but the drug should not be expected to re-start breathing in an apnoeic patient. Similar comments apply to other so-called antagonists such as vanillic acid (Vandid). The best agent for the reversal of narcotic depression is naloxone (Narcan).

(iii) Cases of acute sepsis in the throat and neck — particularly quinsy — should never be given thiopentone. This is not an inherent danger of the drug, but of the production of unconsciousness in such cases by any means whatsoever before an airway has been established (by intubation or tracheostomy under local analgesia).

(iv) Operations on the nose, mouth, and throat should not be performed under thiopentone alone.

(v) The inadvertent injection of the drug into an artery may lead to gangrene of the limb. This accident is particularly likely to occur in a fat patient when one of the veins on the medial side of the antecubital fossa is chosen, often due to the presence of an aberrant ulnar recurrent artery, and is obvious from the sudden intense burning pain in the arm and hand complained of by the patient (a mere 0·5 ml is sufficient). In such circumstances leave the needle in the artery and inject 5 ml of 1% procaine (in preference to other local analgesic agents). Alternatively, papaverine 60 mg in saline, or tolazoline (Priscol) may be injected. A sympathetic block is urgently required to open up the circulation of the limb, which is in profound spasm. If necessary, the intended operation must be postponed while these measures are taken. In some cases it may be advisable to heparinize the patient.

Warning that the accident is likely to occur comes from pulsation transmitted to the needle and a particular brightness of the blood withdrawn into the syringe.

The more frequent accident of injection of thiopentone outside the vein is to be avoided by invariably withdrawing blood into the syringe before injecting. Most small perivenous injections give rise to no serious trouble, but it is wise to view all seriously, and treat by:

(i) the injection of 3–5 ml of a solution of hyaluronidase into the area, and

(ii) the application of heat for 24 hours.

Both measures are intended to improve the local circulation and thus remove the irritant as soon as possible.

Uses

Though 5% solutions of the drug have been used in the past, it is better to choose a 2·5% solution to reduce the hazards of extravascular injections, particularly as litigation is so popular these days. Thiopentone may be employed:

(i) For induction.

(ii) As the sole anaesthetic in short minor operations.

(iii) Combined with another agent, usually nitrous oxide.

(i) *Induction.*

Freely applicable to all fit cases, bearing in mind the contraindications already mentioned. The drug may be given to old patients and ill patients provided a small dose only is administered. A watch on the respiration may be misleading if the circulation time is slow. There is a danger of giving a second dose in the belief that the initial amount has been inadequate, whereas it may not have produced its maximum effect. About 0·1–0·2 g will be found to produce unconsciousness in such cases.

The average patient, however, will require about 0·3–0·4 g of thiopentone, which may be injected quite rapidly. The anaesthetic may then be continued with any other agent, such as trichlorethylene or halothane. After such an induction bear in mind:

(a) The possibility of laryngeal spasm — increase the strength of anaesthetic vapour gently.

(b) The anaesthetic will, paradoxically, transiently lighten as the induction is recommenced with gaseous agents, owing to the diminishing effect of the injected thiopentone.

(c) The respiration may be temporarily depressed. The reservoir bag may be compressed a few times until respiration is recommenced.

(d) You must keep a clear airway. (Again!)

(ii) *As the sole anaesthetic for short minor operations.*

Induction may be performed as outlined above, the needle being kept *in situ* with the left thumb on the hub and the other fingers of the left hand circling the arm. With this grip any sudden movement of the patient will draw the syringe with it; the right hand is free to press the plunger, and to support the jaw if no other help is available.

Once the patient has lost consciousness, as marked by the onset of automatic respiration, the loss of the eyelash reflex, and occasionally a deep yawn, attention must then be concentrated upon the breathing and the injection discontinued if it ceases.

The student often asks, "How do I know when to inject more of the drug?" and the reply is not simple. The occurrence of reflex movements is the surest guide, but these may easily disrupt the anaesthesia and the operation. The respiration is usually so depressed under thiopentone that the character of the breathing is of little use as a sign of anaesthesia. Careful observation of the respiration and a little experience is the answer to the question.

Reflex movement may persist under quite deep thiopentone narcosis, and it is advisable if some painful though short operation is anticipated (e.g., opening a septic pulp infection, removal of a big toenail) for the part to be held by an assistant. This enables the operation to be completed equally satisfactorily without subjecting the patient to a deep anaesthetic with its subsequent prolonged recovery period.

(iii) Combined with another agent.

The student is not advised to attempt narcosis for long operations under thiopentone alone. For any but the shortest procedures it is preferable to use the technique of thiopentone-gas-oxygen anaesthesia.

Once anaesthesia has been established with thiopentone, its continuance with nitrous oxide and oxygen administered in a ratio of 6:2 provides an anaesthetic that is free from anoxia, without marked after-effects, and suitable for operations requiring light surgical anaesthesia. Such an administration may be continued for many hours if necessary, the addition of a little adjuvant anaesthetic to the mixture from time to time assisting in maintaining the patient at the required depth. Trichlorethylene is useful in this role.

This thiopentone-gas-oxygen sequence will be found useful for all minor procedures lasting more than a few minutes — the setting of fractures is a frequent example. At the same time, such a method may be used for longer operations on the superficial structures when the anaesthetist is asked to do little more than keep the patient asleep. It is also the commonest mixture for maintaining light anaesthesia in combination with muscle relaxants, since it has the advantages of being almost non-toxic and non-explosive. The amount of thiopentone required when the drug is followed by nitrous oxide is much less than the amount demanded if the operation were to be performed under thiopentone alone. Conversely, possible anoxia from the administration of nitrous oxide and oxygen is avoided by the larger oxygen percentage made possible by the use of thiopentone.

(iv) *Basal Narcosis*.

There is still a place for basal narcosis in children, especially those who must be subjected to repeated and possibly unpleasant diagnostic or therapeutic procedures (e.g., lumbar puncture, examination of fundi). For this purpose it is administered in a 5% solution in a dosage of 1 g per 20 kg of body weight. The small volume required does not usually have the effect of an enema and the duration of narcosis is brief — two points greatly in its favour. Suppositories and a pre-packaged suspension are available, and have the merit of convenience. The full effects should be manifest in about 20 minutes and will last for about ¾ to 1 hour, though the patient may remain asleep for much longer and during this period must be under supervision.

Other Intravenous Drugs

Methohexitone (Brietal) is perhaps the most important. Like thiopentone it is a barbiturate, so that the general comments made about that drug apply. It is injected in a 1% solution in a dose of about 100 mg for the average adult. Rapid effect and recovery are its main advantages, making it particularly suitable for use in the out-patient and dental departments. It is less irritating to the tissues if injected extravenously, and causes less depression of the cardiovascular system. On the debit side, there is greater liability to jerky muscular movements, hiccup, and coughing.

For completeness, other drugs must be mentioned which are not barbiturates. Propanidid (Epontal) is a eugenol derivative, but used in a similar manner for induction or very brief anaesthesia. There is little hangover effect because of its rapid and complete destruction in the body. It is administered intravenously in a dose of 5–10 mg/kg, but as the solution is rather viscid a larger needle is usually required. It often causes a brief spell of over-breathing followed by an equally brief period of apnoea. Occasionally it causes venous thrombosis at the site of injection.

Althesin may also be encountered as an alternative for induction. It is a mixture of two steroid substances, and like propanidid brings a clear-headed recovery. The recommended dose is 50–60 mg/kg.

Diazepam (see p. 16) is rarely employed as an induction agent but it is widely used for sedation. Indeed, chemically, it is closely related to nitrazepam, used as a narcotic (see p. 17). In a dose of 5–10 mg, which may be repeated, it is particularly valuable for providing sleep during an operation performed under local analgesia or for mild sedation during diagnostic procedures.

Finally, mention must be made of ketamine (Ketalar), which may be given intramuscularly as well as intravenously, an advantage with small children. It is particularly useful for diagnostic and radiotherapeutic procedures in children, having largely replaced rectal thiopentone, or when surgery must be performed in unfavourable circumstances without the benefit of skilled anaesthesia. Involuntary movements not apparently in response to stimulation are common, which limits its usefulness in delicate procedures, e.g., eye surgery or eye examination unless a general anaesthesia is added. Respiratory depression is slight, a rise in blood pressure not uncommon (be careful with the hypertensive patient), and the airway is usually well maintained. It may cause some emergence reactions and hallucinations, which seem more troublesome to adults than to children. It is important to allow a recovery as peaceful as possible and in the patient's own time. Vigorous efforts at arousal only encourage unpleasant reactions. The dose is 10 mg/kg intramuscularly, preferably of a 10% solution, to reduce the total volume, intravenously, 2 mg/kg of a 1% solution is given initially, and can be repeated.

Halothane

Halothane (Fluothane) is a volatile anaesthetic and almost the most expensive. It is a clear, heavy liquid with a smell similar to chloroform. In fact, it resembles chloroform in many ways.

Advantages
(1) Halothane is non-flammable.
(2) It is non-irritant to the respiratory tract and induction is not unpleasant.
(3) Anaesthesia is achieved rapidly and smoothly.
(4) Recovery is similarly rapid.
(5) The masseter muscles relax early and the laryngeal reflexes are depressed, aiding the insertion of an airway or an endotracheal tube.
(6) The fall in blood pressure may be turned to advantage as a means of reducing blood loss.

Disadvantages

(1) There is frequently a marked fall in blood pressure, due mainly to a reduction of cardiac output and partly to peripheral vasodilation. The hypotension is often associated with bradycardia, which should be treated with intravenous atropine 0·6 mg.

(2) Respiratory depression is common and may require assisted ventilation.

(3) Since halothane is such a potent agent, and is effective in small concentrations, it should be administered by a specially calibrated vaporizer (for example, the Fluotec. See p. 64).

(4) It produces marked relaxation of the uterus and may cause post-partum haemorrhage unless used with care.

(5) Good muscular relaxation can be achieved only at the expense of hypotension and serious respiratory depression.

(6) Before anaesthesia has been reached, it has no analgesic properties.

(7) Recovery is sometimes stormy because of rapid recovery without residual analgesia, the patient sensing pain from his wound before consciousness is regained. There may also be marked shivering. To avoid this, a trace of trichlorethylene may be added to the anaesthetic towards the end of the operation.

(8) Halothane in a moist atmosphere corrodes light metals (zinc, tin, aluminium), ruining any moving parts.

(9) There seems little doubt that liver damage may follow halothane anaesthesia. The exact mechanism is uncertain, but as it occurs most commonly after repeated administrations a sensitivity reaction is suspected. Clinically, the condition resembles virus hepatitis, from which it is difficult to distinguish. On biochemical and histological evidence, it can be clearly differentiated from most other causes of jaundice. Statistical evidence for this complication is questioned, and other possible causative factors are so frequent, that it is unwise to be too dogmatic explaining it.

(10) Because of (9) above, halothane should not be administered to anyone who has received a previous halothane anaesthetic within the last four weeks. It is incumbent on the anaesthetist to ask a specific question about previous anaesthetics.

Uses

(1) Halothane administered with nitrous oxide and oxygen may be used for any operation not requiring profound muscular relaxation. It is more powerful than trichlorethylene.

(2) For induction before the administration of the more irritant vapour of ether.

(3) As an adjuvant, mainly to achieve controlled hypotension.

(4) Other more specialized uses, as for thoracic surgery.

The *particular disadvantages* may restrict the use of this drug for the inexperienced anaesthetist. But if certain safeguards are observed:

  (i) atropine premedication to reduce the vagal effect on the heart

 (ii) use of a calibrated vaporizer, keeping the halothane concentration between $0.5-2\%$

(iii) avoidance fo closed-circuit anaesthesia (economical, but not for the tyro)

(iv) a careful and continuous watch on respiration and blood pressure

the dangers can be much reduced.

Halothane must be treated with great respect. Nevertheless, the smooth and rapid induction followed by a ready control of the depth of anaesthesia are great advantages. If used intelligently and with an understanding of its effects, a simple mixture of nitrous oxide, oxygen, and halothane is a safe and reasonable choice in a wide variety of procedures.

Trichlorethylene

A liquid with a vapour heavier than air, useful for the production of analgesia and light anaesthesia but useless for the establishment of deep anaesthesia. Because the smell of trichlorethylene is similar to that of chloroform, the manufacturers add a blue dye to assist in its recognition.

Advantages

  (i) Trichlorethylene is a safe anaesthetic, but there do appear to have been a small, but definite, number of cases of primary cardiac failure caused by the drug.

 (ii) It is pleasant to inhale.

(iii) It is non-flammable.

(iv) It produces little post-operative nausea or disturbance.
(v) It produces a high degree of analgesia without loss of consciousness.
(vi) Analgesia is carried into the post-operative period, often reducing the need for additional pain relief.

Disadvantages

(i) Trichlorethylene is suitable only for the maintenance of *light* anaesthesia.
(ii) The drug is not always simple to administer, as tachypnoea may occur. Avoiding an overdose may be difficult, even with calibrated vaporizers, some patients seeming unduly sensitive to its effect on respiration. The tachypnoea is from disturbance of the Hering-Breuer reflex, expiration occurring before inspiration is complete and vice versa. The tidal exchange falls until it may nearly approach the dead space volume, to cause carbon dioxide retention and hypoxia. Both are potent causes or aggravating features of cardiac irregularities.
(iii) Transient cardiac arrhythmias occasionally occur, though these have never proved detrimental to the patient. (Tachycardia, extrasystoles, and auricular fibrillation are the most common, in that order.)
(iv) The drug requires some sort of vaporizing apparatus for its use.
(v) It cannot be used in the closed circuit apparatus for fear of decomposition of the vapour with the production of nerve palsies.
(vi) Trichlorethylene is excreted slowly from the body and recovery may be delayed.

Particular dangers

There appear to be none apart from those in the preceding paragraph, provided the recommended concentrations are not exceeded.

Uses

Trichlorethylene is of considerable use, if properly given, for producing a light anaesthesia for superficial operations, and the combination of the drug with a spinal or local analgesic or with a muscle relaxant has made it of use in abdominal operations. Moreover, its non-irritant qualities stamp it as a useful drug for the induction of anaesthesia, once unconsciousness has been established with nitrous oxide or thiopentone and before the administration of the more pungent vapour of ether.

The student can easily master the technique of trichlorethylene administration for light surgical anaesthesia by carefully observing the following rules:

(i) Establish the narcosis with thiopentone.

(ii) Add trichlorethylene to the gas-oxygen mixture administered during the operation *in the smallest quantity possible*. An overdose of the drug invariably leads to tachypnoea.

(iii) Should tachypnoea occur, reduce the concentration. If this fails, immediately discontinue the drug, substituting some other agent if necessary.

(iv) Shut off the trichlorethylene about the middle of the operation, if the patient is satisfactorily anaesthetized, in order that the long excretion period shall be turned to an advantage in its continuing the anaesthetic.

Trichlorethylene has too low a volatility to be employed without some form of inhaler. It may be used in the usual vaporising bottle in a semi-closed apparatus, or better in the less coarse and smaller Goldman inhaler. Since the concentrations from these are largely guesswork, the calibrated Tritec has obvious advantages.

For the use of trichlorethylene in obstetrics see p. 131.

Ether

A liquid with a vapour heavier than air, a potent anaesthetic which may be used for all types of surgery.

Advantages

(i) Ether is safe, and apparently simple to administer, attributes that demand its continued use in teaching schools despite the occasional opponents to the drug found therein.

(ii) It is, and probably always will be, the ideal agent for learning the classical signs of anaesthesia.

(iii) Ether has little if any toxic action on the heart. An overdose of ether is marked by cessation of respiration, but, unless anoxia is allowed to develop, a finger placed on the pulse finds the heart beating unimpaired. Only a gross overdose, that can be introduced with the use of artificial respiration, will lead to failure of the circulation.

(iv) Relaxation produced by this agent is satisfactory for all abdominal procedures.

(v) Ether is an excellent anaesthetic for administration to children, old people, and the ill.

Disadvantages

(i) Ether possesses a pungent smell and disagreeable taste, rendering its inhalation by the conscious patient unpleasant and leaving an offensive flavour after the administration of large quantities.

(ii) The vapour is highly irritant to the upper respiratory tract, and causes excessive secretion. Ether cannot, however, be blamed for the incidence of post-operative "chests", which show no connexion with the anaesthetic drug employed.

(iii) Induction with ether by itself is slow and unpleasant for the patient, unless assisted by a little of some more powerful and less irritant vapour, such as halothane. Without such assistance it is difficult to produce smooth, untroubled anaesthesia with ether, despite its very real advantage of safety and simplicity.

(iv) Ether is a flammable liquid and vapour.

Particular danger

Explosion risk. Ether is a flammable drug which should never be used with diathermy or cautery or anywhere near a naked flame, a point which limits its value for domicilliary obstetrics. Nor can it be used for bronchoscopy, through danger of ignition from the instrument's bulb, unless a fibre optic system is used. A less obvious but equally serious source of ignition is static electricity. Defective electrical equipment may cause an explosion even some distance from the patient, because a high concentration of ether vapour (as from somebody dropping a bottle of it) is much heavier than air and spreads across the theatre floor. If diathermy is insisted upon during ether administration the drug must be cut off completely at least 10 minutes before granting the surgeon permission to use his apparatus, assuming the patient is breathing sufficiently to reduce the concentration of ether in his body.

Ether/air mixtures are less ignitable and their consequences less violent than those of ether/oxygen or ether/nitrous oxide/oxygen, which are dangerously explosive. The use of ether/air, with which you should be familiar, may on occasion present less of an hazard than the use of a non-flammable agent with which you are not. It is comforting to remember that no explosion has ever been reported using an open system with air as the carrier gas.

Uses

Ether is eminently suitable for the inexperienced administrator called upon to anaesthetize for an abdominal operation. The relaxation provided is good and relatively unaccompanied by danger to the patient.

Do not be afraid of administering a reasonably large quantity of ether for an abdominal operation, particularly if it is being performed upon the upper abdomen (e.g., for perforated duodenal ulcer). Once induction has been completed, the amount of ether vapour delivered to the patient may be steadily increased until the respiration has become entirely abdominal and is diminishing in amplitude. If an overdose should be inadvertently given, then prompt recourse to artificial respiration with pure oxygen or air will leave the patient entirely unaffected.

Large quantities of ether in prolonged operations are neither ideal nor the expert's choice. But ether is one of the safest anaesthetics if not necessarily the simplest to administer elegantly. So if in doubt choose ether.

Where a calibrated vaporizer is available, about 15% is needed to produce surgical anaesthesia though 7–8% would be adequate for maintenance. 4% is just sufficient to keep a patient asleep.

Muscle Relaxants

Curare, which was originally used as an arrow poison by the native tribes of South America, produces a widespread paralysis of muscles by interfering with the normal action of acetylcholine at the neuromuscular junction. With the aid of curare, therefore, an abdominal operation can be performed under light anaesthesia, with benefit to the patient. For practical purposes all the muscles in the body may be taken to be paralysed equally, and it may be assumed that if the surgeon is satisfied with the relaxation the respiration will be inadequate. The anaesthetist must therefore always be ready to substitute the patient's natural respiration by squeezing the reservoir bag; and he must judge the amount and timing of his dose of curare so that the patient is breathing adequately when he leaves the theatre. Fortunately, neostigmine is an antidote to many of the relaxant drugs, and may be used to cancel the mistimed dose.

These points illustrate the main dangers of the muscle-relaxant drugs. Although the student sees them used freely in the operating theatres of his hospital it is inadvisable for him to use them without supervision. He will find he can get himself into quite enough trouble with the old-established agents, however tempting it looks to produce ideal surgical conditions within a few moments by a simple intravenous injection. Though intubation is not necessary for artificial ventilation, it is unwise to paralyse a patient unless you feel confident of your ability to perform this manoeuvre in case of difficulty.

Curare is given in doses of 15–18 mg, takes 2–3 minutes to exert its full effect, and lasts for about 45 minutes.

Gallamine (Flaxedil), the first synthetic curare-like drug, lasts only half an hour and is given in a dose of 80–120 mg.

Pancuronium (Pavulon) is a recent synthetic addition to this group of drugs, and chemically has a steroid structure. It is used in doses of about 6 mg, acting rather more quickly than curare but lasting about the same time. It has little effect on the pulse (whereas gallamine causes tachycardia) or blood pressure, and does not seem guilty of liberating histamine (as does curare on occasions).

Alcuronium (Alloferin) is a chemical relative of pancuronium, with the advantage of swifter paralysis of shorter duration. It may be conveniently used for intubation yet remain effective for some twenty minutes — ideal for such short procedures as laparoscopy. The comparable dose is 12–15 mg.

Suxemethonium (Scoline) has a profound but ultra-short action. In doses of 50–75 mg, it lasts for 3–4 minutes only. It causes a characteristic generalized muscular fibrillation before paralysis. Though probably unrelated to this, many patients who receive suxemethonium suffer from postoperative muscular pains. These seem to be severest in the ambulant patient, and can be most distressing. Unlike the other relaxant drugs, suxemethonium is not antagonized by neostigmine; indeed, its action may be augmented. This variation is related to the different ways in which drugs act. The "curare-like" drugs are competitive blockers but suxemethonium is a depolarizing agent.

Neostigmine is given intravenously as an antidote to the competitive blockers. It must be injected slowly, never faster than 1 mg/minute, until muscle paralysis has been reversed completely. The dose needed may be 1·25–5·0 mg, depending on the amount of muscle relaxant given and when it was administered. Neostigmine does, however, produce effects other than reversal of curarization. It causes bradycardia, stimulation of mucous secretion in the respiratory tract and contraction of the gut. It is necessary therefore to counteract these effects by the preliminary injection of atropine — usually 1·0 mg intravenously five minutes before the neostigmine — even though atropine was given as premedication.

Controlled Hypotension

All general anaesthetics tend to reduce the blood pressure. So does premedication, particularly if this includes a phenothiazine drug. In addition, deliberate reduction of haemorrhage during surgery may be achieved by:

(1) Local ischaemia from the infiltration of dilute solutions of adrenalin.

(2) Extensive spinal or extradural analgesia, which will block the sympathetic pathways.

(3) The intravenous injection of ganglion blocking agents such as the methonium compounds and trimetaphan (Arfonad). Trimetaphan is used as an intravenous drip, and as the action of the drug is usually brief the hypotension produced is more controllable. As an alternative, but used in a similar fashion to trimetaphan, sodium nitroprusside is becoming increasingly popular.

(4) The use of fairly high concentrations of halothane, usually associated with intermittent positive pressure respiration.

Methods (2), (3) and (4) cause vasodilatation with a normal circulating blood volume, a wholly different situation from the hypotension which follows loss of blood. The patient must always be postured with care to reduce the hydrostatic pressure at the operation site, bearing in mind the circulatory demands of the brain. Indeed, under general anaesthesia posture alone may produce a relatively dry surgical field. A clear airway and adequate ventilation are necessary safeguards, and remember that a rise in carbon dioxide tension (a consequence of failing to observe this safeguard) tends to cause a rise in blood pressure. Controlled hypotension has undeniable risks, mainly from impaired cerebral or cardiac circulation, and should be used only by the expert and only when absence of bleeding is not just desirable but imperative. It may be a valuable adjunct to anaesthesia, but is never justified merely as a means of making an operation easy for the surgeon.

Cyclopropane

A non-irritant, powerful, highly explosive, and expensive gas, the latter property demanding its use in the closed circuit apparatus. It is a powerful respiratory depressant and may cause cardiac arrythmias. Though it may be used for most surgical procedures the technique is not simple. It is less popular than it was, and its use is not recommended to the student.

Chloroform

A classical, powerful, non-flammable agent. Though of use in primitive conditions, it should not normally be given because of the danger of primary cardiac failure — a hazard not easily guarded against. Its particular properties can be readily obtained by consulting any textbook of pharmacology[1].

Methoxyflurane

Methoxyflurane (Penthrane) is a halogenated ether with a high boiling point and a low vapour pressure. Thus concentrations of no more than 4% can be administered. It has two great advantages: it is non-flammable and provides excellent analgesia. Induction is slow, though the vapour is not unpleasant to breathe.

Recent reports have shown that prolonged administrations may be followed by renal damage. This is indicated by a high output of urine with a low fixed specific gravity, often persisting for several weeks, but usually with ultimate recovery. Headaches and dizziness are not uncommon, and may be suffered by the administrator as well as the patient.

---

[1] Chloroform has the distinction of being the only anaesthetic to figure in a murder trial. In 1886 a grocer named Edwin Bartlett was found dead in his Pimlico flat, and chloroform was later recovered from his stomach. As his wife, the beautiful Adelaide Bartlett, was the only person with him on the evening of his death and had a few days before persuaded a young Methodist minister, her paramour, to buy her some chloroform, she was promptly indicted for murder at the Old Bailey. The case turned on her abilities as an amateur anaesthetist. Could she have chloroformed her husband in his sleep? The jury hesitatingly acquitted her, to the delight of several thousand admirers outside in Newgate Street and Sir James Paget in nearby Barts, who ungallantly suggested that now the verdict was out the young woman should in the interests of medical science explain exactly how she did it.

Carbon Dioxide

A cylinder of carbon dioxide may be attached to an anaesthetic apparatus and is of use for:

(i) Stimulating the respiration during induction. One litre per minute temporarily added to the 2·6 oxygen gas mixture is adequate, and the induction is thus accelerated.

(ii) Before the nasal passage of endotracheal tubes "blind", now rarely attempted.

(iii) For the relief of hiccough, which occurs occasionally during operations. Add about 0·5 litre of carbon dioxide per minute to the gas mixture.

(iv) Carbon dioxide is a powerful respiratory stimulant and may be used as such provided that:

    (a) the muscles of respiration are not paralysed

    (b) the respiratory centre is capable of responding to the stimulus. Usually, however, during a period of depressed respiration from whatever cause, the patient suffers from an excess rather than a deficiency of carbon dioxide.

Too much carbon dioxide will poison the respiratory centre. Remember that this gas is present in the normal exhalation without addition from a cylinder, and accumulates in a patient wherever there is

    (a) respiratory obstruction

    (b) inadequate respiratory exchange

    (c) exhausted soda lime in a closed circuit apparatus

    (d) rebreathing as a result of inadequate total gas flow in an open circuit

    (e) increase in dead space from faulty apparatus (jammed valves, detachment of delivery tube in a coaxial tube, etc.).

Anaesthetics and the Anaesthetist

The newer anaesthetic agents, particularly halothane and methoxyflurane, have revealed the hazards to which anaesthetists may be exposed from the agents they handle. We have also been made to realize that gases vented in the operating theatre may have undesirable effects on others working in the contaminated atmosphere — even nitrous oxide may be harmful — but unfortunately, we do not yet know what sort of concentrations may be dangerous.

Headache and dizziness have been reported frequently. Pregnancies suffer an increased incidence of abortions, minor congenital deformities and a higher percentage of female births. It is clear that the possibilities of teratogenicity must be investigated further.

Liver damage has been reported in anaesthetists, also conjunctivitis and cardiac arrhythmias.

So try not to poison yourself by breathing exhaust gases and vapours unnecessarily. Use those safety devices available — ducted vents, charcoal adsorbers, etc.

CHAPTER 6

Apparatus

All that is necessary for the administration of an anaesthetic gas is a cylinder of the compressed agent, a tap to control the flow, and a piece of tubing leading to the patient's face. During the last century, however, this simple plan has become refined in the following respects:

(1) The provision of reducing valves on the gas cylinders, by means of which the high intracylinder pressure—about 2,000 lb/sq in (140 kg/cm^2, or 133 bar) for oxygen, 750 lb/sq in (50 kg/cm^2, or 50 bar) for nitrous oxide, both at 15°C—is reduced to a more convenient level.

(2) An accurate tap allowing a measured amount of the gas per minute to be administered to the patient. This may be incorporated in a mixing chamber permitting a definite percentage of nitrous oxide in oxygen to be delivered.

(3) A reservoir bag from which the patient takes each inhalation.

(4) A face-mask or nose-piece. This ensures the mixture is inhaled unadulterated with outside air, and is equipped with a valve for the release of each exhalation.

The only essential piece of apparatus for the inhalation of the liquid anaesthetics is a piece of gauze or similar material upon which the drug may be poured for vaporization. A dome-shaped wire frame mask (Schimmelbusch, or similar type), and the securing of an air-tight fit round the nose and mouth with a Gamgee pad are early elaborations of the simple apparatus which are in use today when more complicated equipment is not available. A later step was the introduction of inhalers, of which Clover's[1] ether inhaler enjoyed the longest and most

---

[1] Joseph Clover (1825–1882) succeeded John Snow as Victorian England's leading anaesthetist. He maintained the same scientific and practical approach to a young subject that might easily have suffered from ignorance, over-enthusiasm, and superstition.

deserved popularity. With these instruments the anaesthetic could be more economically and conveniently administered.

Present-day anaesthetic apparatus results from the marriage of the systems for the administration of gaseous and volatile agents. The *continuous flow semi-open machine* is found in hospitals all over the country. This is a simple type of apparatus to use, and will be afforded prominence in this chapter as being the most likely equipment that the student will be required to operate.

The continuous flow apparatus consists essentially of cylinders of compressed nitrous oxide and oxygen equipped with reducing valves, from which the gases flow through control taps to flowmeters, through further taps over the surface of the liquid anaesthetics, and thence to the patient.

The Cylinders

The usual equipment is one working cylinder and one reserve each of nitrous oxide and oxygen, and sometimes a single cylinder of carbon dioxide. Always change an empty cylinder as soon as it is exhausted, and always be certain that the reserve cylinder is, in fact, full. Cylinders, once empty, must be clearly marked and stored away from the full ones. The cylinders are locked to the apparatus in a metal yoke with two pins fitting holes on the cylinder head of one particular gas only. Each cylinder is painted according to a standard code of colours:

Oxygen	Black, with white shoulders
Nitrous oxide	Blue
Entonox	Blue, with blue and white quartered shoulders
Cyclopropane	Orange
Carbon dioxide	Grey

The cylinders are equipped with

Reducing Valves

The valves are not interchangeable. They consist essentially of a spring-loaded diaphragm to counteract the intracylinder pressure, and must be promptly repaired if faulty or noisy. The oxygen valve always carries a *pressure gauge*, informing the anaesthetist of the amount of oxygen remaining in the cylinder. In the case of nitrous oxide, which is in the form of liquid in the cylinder, such a gauge would give no indication of the contents until the cylinder were almost exhausted. Metal leads carry the gases to their separate flowmeters.

Flowmeters

These are customarily arranged in a bank of two or more on the anaesthetic trolley, and lead into a common channel in which the gases mix.

The **rotameter** is the most common type of flowmeter on anaesthetic machines today. It is highly accurate, having duralumin bobbins spinning in the gas flow clear of the walls of a tapered glass tube, so avoiding errors from friction. These bobbins are read from their flat tops, and the rotameter is calibrated in 100 ml per minute or in litres per minute.

The rotameter is a "variable area — constant pressure drop" type of meter, the variable area being the ring between the bobbin and the walls of the tapered glass tube.

Access of gases to these flowmeters is by needle valves under the anaesthetist's control.

A **dry bobbin** or a **water sight** flowmeter may be found on oxygen therapy apparatus where no great degree of accuracy is needed.

From the flowmeter the mixed gases pass through a metal tube to which various vaporizing devices may be connected.

Vaporizers

The most usual consists of a sleeve valve which directs part or all of the gas flow into a glass bottle containing the liquid anaesthetic. The strength of the vapour emitted depends on four factors — the surface area of the liquid, the rate of gas flow, the manner in which the gas impinges on the liquid, and the temperature of the liquid. All except the temperature of the liquid can be altered — albeit crudely — by the anaesthetist. He may:

(1) Vary the gas flow from the flowmeters.
(2) Turn the sleeve valve so that more gas enters the bottle.
(3) Depress an adjustable plunger which directs the gas flow closer to the surface of the liquid.
(4) Depress the plunger below the surface of the liquid so that the gas bubbles through it.

As these simple vaporizers cool rapidly during use, the vapour pressure falls, and it becomes impossible to control the concentration of vapour delivered. As mentioned on p. 50, it is not only helpful but almost essential for the concentration of potent agents like halothane to be metered accurately. Thus, more sophisticated vaporizers incorporating thermocontrol mechanisms are becoming increasingly common. These may be specially calibrated for any anaesthetic agent, but the most usual is the Fluotec for halothane.

As you should think in terms of accurate concentrations instead of using inspired guesswork, the following table of percentages may be helpful.

	Induction of surgical anaesthesia	Maintenance of surgical anaesthesia	"Sleep"
Ether	15	7–8	4
Halothane	3	1·5–2	0·5–1
Trichlorethylene ..	—	1·0–1·5 (light anaesthesia only)	0·5
Methoxyflurane ..	3–4	1	0·3

We now have a mixture of nitrous oxide and oxygen carrying with it a variable amount of volatile agents. The mixture returns to the delivery pipe to reach the patient via

The Magill Semi-open Bag Attachment

This piece of apparatus, first designed by Magill, was intended to allow part of the patient's exhalation to escape into the atmosphere and part to return to the apparatus to mix with the oncoming flow of gases. Thus, some economy of anaesthetic gases was achieved, and a small percentage of the patient's exhaled CO_2 added to each inhalation, depending on the gas flow.

It is recognized today that one of the anaesthetist's primary responsibilities is to eliminate carbon dioxide. Thus, although Magill's apparatus is used, a higher flow of gases (to be on the safe side, roughly equivalent to the patient's minute volume) is delivered through the apparatus to avoid rebreathing.

The apparatus consists of:
(1) A rubber reservoir bag.
(2) A metre of corrugated rubber tubing, of wide bore to preclude obstruction and offer the minimal resistance to respiration.
(3) A face-piece with a spring-loaded expiratory valve.

The apparatus requires a gas-flow of about 8 litres per minute to prevent the accumulation of carbon dioxide, though possibly a more accurate measurement would be provided by the alveolar ventilation. A fall in the gas-flow below this figure will be evident from the increase in depth and rate of the patient's respirations. It is customary to deliver a mixture of six litres of nitrous oxide to two of oxygen per minute, though the proportion of oxygen should be increased if there is any suspicion that hypoxia is occurring to the smallest degree. The expiratory valve should be adjusted as loosely as possible.

The entire machine is usually arranged round a trolley upon which the nurses neatly collect a selection of supplementary apparatus of varying usefulness. The trolley is mounted on anti-static castors, and all the rubber components will be made of anti-static material (indicated by the word "antistatic" or a yellow line), to discourage the formation of static electricity with the possible sequel of an explosion.

The mask may be secured to the unconscious patient's face by a harness, the usual types found in Britain being:

(1) Clausen's. This appliance consists of a Y-shaped perforated rubber strap. A ring bearing three hooks is slipped over the dome of the face-piece and the two short arms of the Y reasonably firmly attached to it across the patient's cheeks. The long arm is loosely hooked across the top of the head.

(2) Connell's. This consists of a headpiece with pairs of rubber loops on either side. The loops slide through metal clips which allow easy adjustment and can be hooked directly to studs on the face mask.

The anaesthetist must take care to avoid pressing the rim of the mask into the patient's eyes.

Before using the anaesthetic apparatus, it must be checked on the following points:

(1) Are the working gas cylinders turned on, and do they contain anything?

(2) Are the reserve cylinders turned off, and are they full? (Tap the nitrous oxide cylinder with a spanner, if you are musically inclined; a full cylinder emits a dull note.)

(3) Are the leads connected to the correct flowmeters? (Highly important in the older machines, but modern apparatus has fixed or non-interchangeable connections designed to prevent accidents.)

(4) Are the flowmeters working?

(5) Are the vaporizing bottles correctly filled? If you did not

fill the bottles yourself turn on the machine and smell each vapour to be certain no mistake has been made.

(6) Is the face-piece rim inflated and is it the correct fit for the patient? (Do *not* try a few on him for size.) Difficulty may be experienced in applying the face-piece firmly to some unconscious patients, particularly edentulous ones, in which case the cheeks should be bunched into the sides of the mask.

(7) Is the surgeon going to use diathermy? If he is, then any flammable agents should be removed from the apparatus and left outside the theatre.

When using this type of machine for induction, turn on the nitrous oxide alone at the rate of some 8–10 litres per minute until unconsciousness has been established, holding the mask above the patient's face and about six inches away. Once the patient is asleep apply the mask firmly to the face, open slightly the control of the vaporizer, and adjust the flow of gases in a ratio of oxygen: nitrous oxide = 2 : 6. It is preferable to administer a non-irritant vapour such as trichlorethylene or halothane at this light stage of narcosis, and if ether is used at once it must be given most patiently to avoid reflex coughing and breath-holding. From this point it is simply a matter of increasing the anaesthetic to the concentration required by gently opening the valves with each expiration. The whole process is reviewed in the final chapter.

The Closed Circuit

The closed circuit machine, depending on the principle that CO_2 is absorbed by soda lime, may be used with any anaesthetic except trichlorethylene. It first became popular for economy during the administration of cyclopropane, and its continued use is due partly to habit, since cyclopropane is no longer fashionable, and partly to the misguided belief that a closed circuit apparatus is essential for controlled respiration.

The machine consists of:

(1) A canister of soda lime of proved optimum size and shape.

(2) Unidirectional valves passing each exhalation through the canister.

(3) Two wide bore rubber tubes leading from these valves, through one of which the patient inhales, exhaling into the other.

(4) A gas-tight face-mask, equipped with a valve for releasing too great a pressure in the circuit.

(5) A narrow delivery tube, bringing fresh gases to the face-piece.
(6) A reservoir bag.
(7) A special closed-circuit vaporizing bottle for volatile anaesthetics.

Once the circuit is filled with oxygen and (say) cyclopropane it is necessary to add only:

(1) Oxygen, continuously, at some 300 ml per minute. This replaces the oxygen metabolized by the body (about 250 ml per minute) and that lost by diffusion from the wound and through leaks.
(2) Cyclopropane, intermittently, to increase the depth of anaesthesia when necessary and to replace traces of the gas lost as above.

This system is economical, and has the virtue of preserving the heat and humidity of the patient's exhalations, but suffers from three disadvantages:

(1) The resistance to breathing through soda-lime and a complicated piece of apparatus may be high, making it unsuitable for children.
(2) Soda-lime will become exhausted after 2–3 hours' use, even if intermittent. Unless this use is recorded and the soda-lime changed accordingly, the patient will be poisoned with carbon dioxide.
(3) The concentration of anaesthetic within the circuit tends to rise. This makes it more difficult to achieve a "fine adjustment" in the depth of narcosis than with the semi-open machine.

The closed circuit is, therefore, not as easy for the student to master as the semi-open apparatus, and although a little practice may lead to confident familiarity, it is wiser for the student to use a simple machine. In fact, it is rare for a fully closed circuit to be used today. More usually, a gas flow is established roughly half-way between the basal requirements and the minute volume (i.e., 3–4 litres per minute) and the expiratory valve left partly open. This provides some economy of gases, elimination of carbon dioxide with soda lime, and the use of nitrous oxide in a non-asphyxial concentration, which would be impossible in the true closed circuit.

It is popular with manufacturers at present to disguise these simple pieces of apparatus as complicated machinery, but however constructed and decorated the principle of the equipment is exactly the same despite the difference of price.

Another method of removing carbon dioxide is by unidirectional valves. These are placed next to the face mask or endotracheal tube mount, and ensure that the total expiration is voided to the atmosphere. It follows that the minute volume of gases supplied by the anaesthetic machine must equal that breathed by the patient. The Ruben valve, actuated by springs, or the Mitchell valve, which incorporates opposing magnets, are most commonly used. The Mitchell valve is suitable only for controlled respiration, but the Ruben valve and the valve system built into the O.I.B. (see p. 69) work also with spontaneous respiration. The coaxial (Bain) circuit is increasingly popular. An inner tube of about 5 mm bore delivers fresh gases to the patient's mouth. Exhalation occurs through the lumen of the surrounding corrugated tube, connected to a mounting on the machine which bears a reservoir bag and expiratory valve. This arrangement has the merit of lightness, economy of gases and ensuring proper removal of carbon dioxide. As exhalation passes through a single port, collection and disposal of waste gases is simplified.

Pipelines

Most modern operating theatres and anaesthetic rooms are equipped with piped nitrous oxide and oxygen, obviating the risks of faulty connections and empty cylinders. It may be impossible to check which gas is being delivered, but rigorous examination of the system on installation and non-interchangeable fittings reduce this hazard to a minimum. It is essential, as with cylinder supply, to ensure correct union of leads, particularly after inadvertent disconnection.

The gases are delivered from banks of large cylinders at the usual pressures. After passage through a master valve the gas is reduced to a more workable pressure and distributed to the theatres or wards at 60 lb/sq in (4·5 kg/cm). Automatic switchgear opens a new bank of cylinders as the one in use empties. At the same time a warning light at some strategic point is operated, indicating that the empty cylinders should be replaced as soon as possible. In grander installations, a liquid oxygen tank replaces the bank of oxygen cylinders.

Even with a pipeline supply, all machines should carry a spare oxygen and nitrous oxide cylinder in case of some unexpected fault in the system. Pipelines have the disadvantage of tethering the machine to a boom or wall outlet.

Draw-over Inhalers

An important advantage of the draw-over inhaler is its low resistance to breathing. Inhalers designed to operate with the driving force of gas delivered from a cylinder have entirely different characteristics, and must not be used on the draw-over principle.

In most apparatus a mixture of nitrous oxide and oxygen is used mainly as a vehicle for other anaesthetic vapours, but it would seem more physiological to allow the patient to breathe the gas mixture with which he is most familiar — air. The Oxford Vaporizer was developed on this principle during World War II, to deliver a known percentage of ether in air. Not needing cylinders of gases for vaporizing the ether, it is both economical and portable, and particularly suitable in those parts of the world where cylinders are difficult to supply and the cost of gases high, as well as in warfare.

More recently, the E.M.O. inhaler has been introduced. This inhaler compensates for unavoidable temperature changes (which would otherwise affect the vapour concentration) by a thermo-control which regulates the gas flow through the vaporizing compartment. A separate concertina-type bag with unidirectional valves, known as the O.I.B. unit, is used with the inhaler. The bag fills with air by the force of the expanding coiled spring inside, and manual compression of the bag allows the lungs to be inflated. Thus the bellows unit may be used by itself for artificial respiration.

Apart from economy, portability, and the use of a physiological gas mixture, the other advantages claimed are:
(1) Individual inhalers may be calibrated for any particular volatile anaesthetic agent and measure accurately the concentration of vapour administered.
(2) By the use of air, cyanosis will proclaim inadequate respiration — which would be masked by an oxygen enriched mixture. Nevertheless, oxygen should be added in patients who, for example, are shocked, anaemic, or are suffering from cardiac or respiratory disease.
(3) The technique is suitable for all types of surgery and all patients, with the exception of those suffering from severe cardiac or respiratory diseases.
(4) Simplicity of apparatus means greater safety, and there are no cylinders to run out.
(5) The unidirectional valve system is effective in removing carbon dioxide.

The accurate measurement of vapour with this apparatus allows one to administer either

(a) a conventional anaesthetic with spontaneous respiration at whatever depth desired, or,

(b) a low concentration of vapour which is sufficient to keep the patient asleep while immobility is achieved with a muscle relaxant.

Other draw-over inhalers include: the Oxford miniature vaporizer (modifications of which, calibrated for tricholoroethylene and halothane, are currently in use by the Services); the Halox-air, an induction unit which allows a limited amount of halothane to be used to facilitate an ether anaesthetic; and various inhalers used for obstetric analgesia.

Intermittent Flow Machines

Such apparatus is intended to supply gases only when the patient inspires. They are constructed on the principle that the passage of gas (or oxygen) into a reservoir bag automatically cuts off the flow of the gas: exhaustion of the reservoir by the patient's own inspiration opens the inlet for the refilling of the bag. This mechanism is incorporated in some machines for nitrous oxide/oxygen anaesthesia in dentistry. There is a control on this apparatus for mixing any percentage of nitrous oxide with oxygen. Such equipment is becoming rare, but may be encountered for some years to come until existing apparatus grows unusable and has to be replaced.

Suction Apparatus

Your suction apparatus is just as important as your anaesthetic machine.

Whatever the motive power of this apparatus, it should be capable of achieving a negative pressure of 400 mm Hg. Of greater importance is its ability to displace a given volume of air per minute. In addition to the usual installed suction or electric pump, a mobile unit (Oxford O_2/Injector Sucker) is available, worked by a cylinder of oxygen and a Venturi jet. Even more portable, and of value for domicilliary or emergency use, are the foot-operated Cape (British) or Ambu (Danish) pumps.

Ventilators

Ventilators of varying complexity are essential equipment for the anaesthetist. Driven by electricity, gas pipe-lines or compressors, they provide mechanical artificial respiration, replacing the rhythmic manual compression of a breathing bag. Their virtue is a reliable, predetermined pattern of respiration, for as long as may be necessary. Apart from maintaining controlled respiration for the anaesthetized patient in the operating theatre, this function may be applied whenever respiratory insufficiency threatens — poisoning, neurological or respiratory diseases, chest and head injuries, or post-operatively, especially after thoracic or cardiac surgery. Death often results from inadequate ventilation rather than the original condition.

As a ventilator replaces normal spontaneous breathing, it must be able to vary the volume and the rate at which gases enter the lungs, to suit the patient and his condition. This may be achieved either by pre-setting the pressure of the gases to be reached in the airway, or by pre-setting the volume of gases which will be delivered. Most mechanical ventilators fall into one or other group (with a confusing array of trade names). Cycling of the machine may be effected also by volume, pressure, or by the introduction of an electronic or other timing device. This usually means varying the rate of the inspiratory and expiratory phases, which alter the wave pattern (as shown by plotting gas pressures against time).

Note that artificial ventilation reverses the pattern of normal inspiration. Instead of air being drawn into the lungs by negative pressure created by enlarging the thoracic cavity, gases are forced into the lungs by positive pressure. The intra-thoracic pressures are altered, reversing the normal pressure gradient by which venous blood returns to the heart. So there is more to a ventilator than simply turning it on. It is essential that you should have an easy familiarity with all aspects of one particular machine before using it. Ventilators are referred to loosely as life-support systems. They can be. They can also kill if faulty or used wrongly. It is always important to remember the care of the unconscious patient and all it entails (p. 94, et seq.).

CHAPTER 7

Endotracheal Anaesthesia

Constant success in the technique is born of patience and practice, with gentleness and concentration as godparents. Success is not simply a matter of inserting a tube in the trachea, however difficult that may be, but in doing so without trauma or post-operative discomfort to the patient and in a reasonable time.

Indications

The number of indications for endotracheal anaesthesia vary with the skill of the intubator. This, too, is related to his skill as an anaesthetist, since a sufficient degree of muscular relaxation, together with the abolition of the relevant reflexes, are essential ingredients for success. However, the use of muscle relaxants, and in particular the ultra-short acting suxemethonium have revolutionized our attitude toward intubation. On the one hand they provide ideal conditions under which a tube may be passed quickly, easily, and with the least trauma. On the other, the necessity of maintaining artificial respiration throughout the course of an operation makes intubation advisable so that

(a) the airway is guaranteed — an essential in artificial respiration; and

(b) the stomach is not inflated at the same time as the lungs.

Apart from anaesthetists' fondness for employing endotracheal tubes whenever muscle relaxants are to be used, the following indications may be listed:

(1) The original and still one of the most important uses of the technique is when the surgeon wishes to operate upon the head or face. The operation would otherwise be a battle for possession of the nose between him and the anaesthetist, a struggle fought out on a sterile field.

(2) Endotracheal anaesthesia is of equal advantage in E.N.T.

72

and dental surgery, enabling the anaesthetist not only to provide an uninterrupted airway despite the surgeon's manipulations, but by use of a throat pack round the tube to seal off the trachea from blood finding its way into the pharynx.

(3) When the patient is in a position that makes it difficult to maintain a clear airway (e.g., prone, steep Tredelenburg).

(4) When there is the possibility of secretions having to be removed from the bronchial tree during the operation (e.g., in patients with bronchiectasis).

(5) When an airway cannot be guaranteed otherwise. This may be when anatomical or pathological conditions interfere with the respiratory tract, or (for instance) an emergency at night when the anaesthetist must perform other duties such as the setting up of a transfusion.

(6) In upper abdominal operations where muscle relaxants are not being used, but where quiet respiration is demanded.

(7) To protect the lower respiratory tract from the inhalation of vomit in patients who may have a full stomach.

(8) To provide a route to the lower respiratory tract for the removal by suction of secretions or vomit caused by any condition, apart from anaesthesia (e.g., head injuries, poisoning, drowning, neurological diseases). The doctor may find ample justification in this for time spent learning the art of intubation.

(9) An extension and combination of (3) (5) (7) and (8) for patients in an intensive care unit. It is often used on such patients as a route for intermittent positive pressure ventilation, which it is now realized may be given in this way for several days. The reduction in dead space is an advantage in spontaneous respiration too.

Contraindications

All the contraindications to intubation are relative, and lack of skill on the part of the anaesthetist is perhaps the most important.

Techniques

There are three means of inserting a tube into the laryngeal opening:

(1) Under direct vision with a laryngoscope, requiring the abolition of reflexes and a degree of muscular relaxation which can be given only by deep narcosis, extensive local analgesia, the muscle relaxants, or a combination of methods. The use of a laryngoscope may give rise to trauma in the hands of the inexperienced, but if good conditions are provided the risk is slight.

(2) Nasal intubation with direct vision. The tube is inserted through the nose, but its final entry into the larynx is visualized by a laryngoscope and may in fact by assisted by the use of Magill forceps.

(3) "Blind" intubation through the nose, which should be practised only by the expert.

Naturally, certain cases must be intubated through the nose, but oral intubation is generally the rule.

Apparatus

(1) Endotracheal tubes

Magill tubes of red rubber and more recently of plastic are made in several sizes and should be suitably cut down to provide a long curve for nasal intubation and a short curve for introduction through the mouth. Discard all limp tubes, and those losing their curve—faults which may result from old age, faulty sterilization, or storage. The correct length of tube may be roughly estimated by doubling the distance from the patient's ear to his nostrils. The sizing of tubes follows a standard, referring to the diameter of the lumen in millimetres rather than to a totally arbitrary scale. For oral intubation, a 10 tube is usually suitable for male adults and 8–9 for females. For nasal intubation, one or two sizes smaller will be needed.

Before using the selected tube make sure that no dry blood clot or other material obstructs the lumen, and attach it firmly to the metal or plastic adaptor.

Besides the usual plain tubes, others are available with an inflatable cuff attached to their lower end. When blown up with air these make an airtight seal with the wall of the trachea, which avoids leakage of gas during artificial respiration and prevents secretions or blood from entering the lower respiratory tract.

Mention should be made of the Oxford tubes. These are for oral intubation only, and are bent almost to a right angle to fit the normal curve of the oropharynx. The curved portion is thickened so that kinking is impossible, a great advantage with infants and during neurosurgical operations where the head is in some unusual position. Although insertion is usually easy, a flexible guide—a gum elastic bougie does very well—may simplify matters. It is worth remembering that whatever type of tube is used, this "trick" of sliding tube over introducer can be invaluable in a difficult intubation. This is particularly so with armoured tubes, which are usually made by dipping a spiral of nylon into latex, giving them incompressibility but leaving them "floppy". They are used where there is risk of kinking an ordinary tube.

(2) The laryngoscope

For direct intubation. There are two types in common use:
 (i) **Magill's,** consisting of a straight metal blade in the form of a half-cylinder, the distal end flattened and bearing a lamp.
(ii) **Macintosh's,** a curved illuminated flat blade, ridged at one side.

Magill's laryngoscope is used to lift the epiglottis forward from behind, so exposing the opening of the larynx. Macintosh's is designed to draw the epiglottis forward from in front (the vallecula). As the area to which this laryngoscope is applied is not, like the posterior surface of the epiglottis, in the direct afferent path of the laryngeal reflex, Macintosh's instrument may be used at a lighter plane of anaesthesia than Magill's and should give rise to less laryngeal spasm. A further advantage is the "open side" which leaves more room in the mouth and thus allows the glottis to be observed during the introduction of the tube. (With the C-shaped laryngoscope blade, the advancing tube often obscures the view of the cords.) The recent fibre-light system, with battery and light source in the handle, offers fewer connections and greater reliability. The illumination is improved but the instrument remains the same.

(3) Magill's forceps

are useful for directing a nasal tube into the trachea under direct vision.

(4) Throat packs

are rolls of bandage soaked in saline and wrung out, placed gently in the pharynx to prevent blood entering the trachea and providing a reasonably airtight fit. If you insert a pack *remember to remove it before withdrawing the tube*. Leave one end of the pack hanging from the mouth as a reminder. If impractical (in dental and some plastic operations) mark the patient's forehead and notes in an easily recognizable manner.

(5) **Lubricants for the tubes.** Choice may be made from:
(i) Water-soluble jelly such as K.Y., suitable for all cases and essential when a cough reflex is required immediately after operation, as in E.N.T. surgery.
(ii) Analgesic jelly, which anaesthetizes the larynx and enables an endotracheal tube to be tolerated under a light plane of anaesthesia without reflex coughing.[1]

The commonest in use today are all preparations incorporating 2 per cent lignocaine. Only the lower third of the tube should be lubricated.

(6) **Local analgesics.** Lignocaine 4% is the most popular. These drugs may be employed for preliminary "cocainization" of the larynx, either under direct vision through a laryngoscope or "blind" by means of a laryngeal spray. Cocaine 4% causes vasoconstriction of the mucous membrane also, and is therefore of particular benefit before nasal intubation. Some anaesthetists use local analgesia before every intubation, but tubes may be passed satisfactorily without this preliminary step. It is important to keep a watch on the total amount of local analgesic solution sprayed into the larynx and trachea. It is dangerously easy to exceed a safe quantity in an attempt to produce perfect analgesia.

Technique of Direct Vision Intubation

It is worth while practising this on any patient who may be sufficiently under the influence of muscle relaxants or deep surgical anaesthesia that he will not respond to the manoeuvre. You may never become a professional anaesthetist, but intubation can be a life-saving measure in many emergencies, both in the casualty department and in the wards.

---

[1] This case is not only genuine but was recounted to no less an audience than the Royal Society of Medicine. At a small hospital in the home counties visited once weekly by a London E.N.T. surgeon, the nursing staff were both alarmed and intrigued by a complete aphonia marring the otherwise immaculate recovery of one of his tonsillectomies. By the time the unusual sequel was discovered both the tonsillectomist and his anaesthetist had stepped into their respective Rolls and were on their way to Harley Street. There was nothing to be done, therefore, until the following visit, when the surgeon rapidly cured the complaint by removing an endotracheal tube, freed from its adaptor, that lay snugly concealed in the patient's nose. Magill tubes are indeed well tolerated without chemical aid.

The essentials are as follows:

(1) **The pillow.** Under the patient's head, with the edge under the shoulders.

(2) **Depth of narcosis.** Never attempt direct intubation unless the patient is in a stage of surgical anaesthesia deep enough to allow complete flaccidity of the jaw muscles and to obtund the laryngeal reflex. Never attempt this method under thiopentone anaesthesia alone.

If the patient is under the influence of muscle relaxants, remember that he is not breathing. If for any reason you run into difficulties and are unable to accomplish your intubation quickly, you must be prepared to inflate the lungs with oxygen and try again after a few moments' rest, keeping a watch on the patient's colour and pulse.

(3) **Positioning the patient.** Remember the direction of the trachea, and that the angle formed by the mouth and pharynx must be converted into a straight line.

(4) **The laryngoscope.**
(i) Magill's: Open the mouth with the right hand, keeping the thumb on the two upper incisors and the forefinger on the lower lip. This position ensures that any condemnable levering that may occur at least does not result in broken upper teeth, and that the lower lip is not nipped between the teeth and the laryngoscope blade.

Insert the blade, keeping the tongue behind the curve. The first landmark is the uvula, which should be brought squarely into the field of vision. Then alter the line of the blade to a more horizontal position and advance it to bring the epiglottis into view. Slip the blade behind the epiglottis and draw the structure forward to expose the laryngeal opening. By this time you should have lowered your own head almost to the level of the patient's. The tube may now be slipped through the glottis.

The metal connecting piece on the tube must lie between the teeth to prevent the airway becoming obstructed should biting occur. If no metal connection is in use, slip an airway alongside the tube to act as a bite block.

(ii) The use of Macintosh's laryngoscope requires the technique to be modified as follows:
(a) A pillow should be bunched under the occiput so that the head is well flexed. This shortens the distance between the lips and the glottis.

(*b*) Even though the instrument may be passed under lighter narcosis than Magill's, the masseters must be flaccid to avoid force in inserting the laryngoscope into the mouth.

(*c*) The blade is placed anterior to the epiglottis, which is drawn forward to expose the larynx, and the curved tube is inserted therein.

(*d*) The blade should be introduced slightly to the right hand side of the mouth and the tongue pushed over to the left. If the blade is introduced in the midline the tongue will curl round the open side of the blade and obstruct the view.

The student should realize some of the

Dangers of Endotracheal Anaesthesia

(1) Damage to the larynx. To be avoided by gentleness and attempting to intubate only at the point of mid-inspiration or mid-expiration when the patient is breathing on his own, or when the cords are sufficiently relaxed by the use of a muscle relaxant.

(2) Tube entering a bronchus — usually the right. This accident, which is commonest in children, results from too long a tube being used. Its occurrence is proclaimed by failure of the patient to settle down after intubation, with coughing and possible cyanosis. Watch the chest carefully for unequal movement. Whenever in doubt, apply a stethoscope to the chest. Whether the patient is breathing spontaneously or being ventilated artificially, absence of breath sounds on one side will be readily proclaimed. Cure is effected by slightly withdrawing the tube.

(3) Detachment of the tube from the adaptor, followed by its disappearance. Under such circumstances:

  (i) Insert a gag.

  (ii) Open the gag and pick the tube from the pharynx.

  (iii) If the tube cannot be found in the pharynx, it is to be retrieved from the larynx or trachea with laryngoscope or bronchoscope.

(4) Blockage of the tube and the connecting catheter mount (the metal adaptor) by blood, mucous, or foreign bodies.[1] Suction may be helpful, but the vigorous insertion of a suction catheter may dislodge a foreign body into the bronchi. It is often better to change the tube.

---

[1] The range of foreign bodies that have been discovered is sweeping, and includes a cockroach, the lens of an eye after cataract extraction, plastic and metal waste, and a paper towel. It is advisable to check patency before inserting the endotracheal tube into the patient.

(5) Kinking the tube at the teeth or pharynx, leading to total respiratory obstruction.

(6) Irritation or damage to the cords, arytenoid cartilages, or the sub-glottic region by pressure or movement of the endotracheal tube. This is most likely to occur in children, and when a much too large tube has been used. Oedema sufficient to cause respiratory obstruction may sometimes develop and be serious enough to warrant tracheostomy.

(7) In nasal intubation, removal of septal spurs, polyps, etc. from the nose, accompanied by profuse haemorrhage. Similarly, dangerous bleeding can occur if an attempt is made to intubate a patient suffering a disorder associated with abnormal bleeding, e.g., haemophilia. The patient's feet must then be raised to prevent the blood running into the trachea, the pharynx packed off when the tube is finally inserted, and any blood that should have entered the trachea must be removed (see p. 26).

(8) A marked fall in oxygen tension, due to the interruption of ventilation during intubation after a muscle relaxant, to coughing, to breathholding, or even to spasm on extubation. The patient may become cyanosed briefly. This is generally of little significance, but must be avoided in the presence of cardiac disease by careful oxygenation before the manoeuvres are started. Prolonged suction (more than 10 to 20 seconds) down an endotracheal tube will also cause a marked fall in oxygen tension, and must be avoided.

Extubation

Unless there are strong indications to the contrary, the patient should be turned on his side before extubation and remain there until the return of consciousness.

After removing the tube at the end of the operation, be sure the patient continues to breathe. An airway is advisable, and should be inserted *before* the tube is removed for fear of reflex tightening of the masseters in response to the passage of the tube through the pharynx and larynx. Some anaesthetists occasionally leave a nasal tube *in situ* with a safety pin through the protruding end, to be removed when the patient starts coughing in the recovery room or ward.[1] Until the tube is removed, the patient should be under the constant supervision of a responsible person and should, again, be nursed on his side.

[1] The morning after returning a patient thus, an anaesthetist at a small hospital was alarmed to read in the night nurse's report, "Oesophageal feeding was difficult, but three ounces of egg-and-milk were retained despite the patient's lack of co-operation." At another institution the sister withdrew and cut off an inch daily, for drainage.

CHAPTER 8

The Condition of The Patient: Shock

The anaesthetist is obliged to accept the double responsibility of administering the anaesthetic and observing, maintaining, and improving the condition of his patient. Both functions are of equal importance.

Most operations leave the subject remarkably undisturbed, but it is up to you to allow the surgeon to concentrate on his own work by taking all worry about the patient's physical state off his shoulders.

The exact pathology of shock is still unknown. It has been defined as "the inability of the circulation to meet the oxygen needs of the tissues and the removal of their metabolites". Treatment must concentrate on adequate perfusion rather than merely raising the arterial pressure. Excluding temporary episodes of a vasovagal nature, the common causes of shock which the anaesthetist meets are:

(1) Haemorrhage.
(2) Loss of extracellular fluid.
(3) Toxins.
(4) Drug overdose.

The Signs of Shock

When shock is due to blood or fluid loss, as it usually is on the operating table, the signs are:

(1) Fall in the blood pressure.
(2) Rise in the pulse rate.
(3) Pallor.
(4) Sweating.
(5) Coldness of the skin.

In short—shock has occurred when a patient who was previously warm, dry, pink, and with a good pulse, becomes cold, moist, and pale, with a bad pulse.

During the operation these signs must therefore be carefully sought:

(1) **The pulse.**

Observe the patient's pulse as carefully as you were instructed in the medical wards, noting particularly:

    (i) Rate.

    (ii) Volume — indicating the blood pressure.

    (iii) Rhythm — arrhythmias are not uncommon under anaesthesia, but their significance is not always clear.

The pulse may conveniently be observed at:

    (i) The superficial temporal artery — just in front of the tragus.

    (ii) The facial artery — where it crosses the mandible, directly anterior of the masseter.

    (iii) The carotids in the neck — particularly if the pulse is impalpable elsewhere.

    (iv) The radial artery.

    (v) The dorsalis pedis artery — just lateral to the extensor tendon of the big toe. A useful point to take the pulse during operations on the upper half of the body.

In all major operations a sphygmomanometer and stethoscope should be attached to the patient's arm and a ten-minute check of pulse and blood pressure recorded on a chart. The information gained from these observations is valuable, but does not take the place of sound clinical judgment — nor must chart-keeping distract the anaesthetist from his more important duties.

During major surgery, direct arterial monitoring is often advisable. A plastic cannula, introduced through a needle in an artery (usually the radial), is connected by a three-way tap to a monitor — an expensive electronic device or a Tycos gauge. The third limb allows the system to be flushed with heparinized saline when necessary. Not for the student.

(2) **The colour.**

Watch not only for cyanosis but for pallor. This too is first seen in the lobes of the ears.

(3) **The skin.**

Never be afraid of touching your patient to note the presence of any sweating and the approximate skin temperature. In fact, we recommend that you keep in physical contact with your patient throughout any operation.

(4) **Blood loss.**

Always estimate the amount of blood being lost by the patient. It is difficult to form more than a rough idea from the amount on swabs, towels, gowns, and possibly the floor, though the bottle of a suction pump is a more accurate guide. At least you can classify your patient as:

    (i) Bleeding severely.

    (ii) Bleeding moderately.

    (iii) Not bleeding much.

In many instances it is important that an accurate estimate be made of the amount of blood lost. This can be done by weighing the swabs after use and subtracting the weight of an equivalent number of dry, unused swabs. This procedure is the only possible way of keeping a check on blood loss in infants. It is easy to forget how small a baby's circulating volume of blood may be, and how high a proportion of this volume a few blood-soaked swabs may represent.

(5) The operation.

Always keep an eye on what the surgeon is up to.[1] The more vigorous the manipulations of the surgeon, and the longer the operation, the more likely is it that shock will be produced even in a healthy patient unless the onset of the condition is guarded against. Ill patients show the signs of shock earlier. Whether shock occurs or not depends so much on the physique of the patient and the technique of the surgeon and anaesthetist that it is difficult to draw up a list of operations in which the condition is most likely to arise.

Early Signs of Shock

As with every other pathological state, early diagnosis increases the chances of successful treatment. Shock often occurs with great suddenness and presents few warning signs.

Very often pallor and coldness are obvious before the circulation shows signs of failing. A slight drop in the systolic pressure and an increase of a few beats a minute in the pulse rate should always be regarded with suspicion when shock is likely to occur, the pulse and the blood pressure being observed every five minutes thereafter.

---

[1] Unobtrusively, however. Nothing annoys a surgeon more than seeing his anaesthetist flying round the theatre like a septic poltergeist. A good anaesthetist should have the character of a Jeeves: he should exercise a strict but subtle control over his surgeon, anticipate his wants, cool his unwise enthusiasms, and encourage him in despair—but from the background. The anaesthetist should make himself the centre of the theatre only when the surgeon is in difficulties before an audience of his distinguished contemporaries.

Shock due to endotoxins is often heralded by extreme hypotension, fever, and rigors. The skin may be warm and dry at first, only later becoming a bluish grey. Renal failure may follow. With drug overdosage, there is a loss of vascular tone and blood tends to "pool", hypothermia is common, and ventilation is often seriously depressed.

Causes of Shock

The clinical causes of shock in the theatre appear to be:
 (i) Severe haemorrhage.
 (ii) Extensive surgical trauma.
(iii) Prolonged operating time.
(iv) Prolonged deep anaesthesia. Crile's theory is that light anaesthesia predisposes to shock, in that the sensory impulses from the operation site are continually reaching the cortex. The performance of extensive procedures under light anaesthesia, including abdominal and thoracic operations with the aid of muscle relaxants, has thrown discredit on this hypothesis.
 (v) Fluid loss
    (a) blood
    (b) tissue fluid
    (c) exhaled moisture
    (d) sweat.
(vi) Inadequate anaesthesia. In spite of the remarks made above, a patient can undoubtedly be brought to a state of shock by vigorous manipulation, especially of the abdominal contents, performed under inadequate anaesthesia and inadequate curarization.

Prevention of Shock

(i) The administration of as small amount of anaesthetic drug as practicable is a rule applying equally to general, local, and spinal techniques.

(ii) Prevention of as much fluid loss as possible. In this connexion the closed-circuit technique may have some advantage over the open method of administration, but not enough to prejudice your choice of anaesthetic technique.

(iii) Beware of over-heating the patient, and remember that the pre-operative atropine or hyoscine will reduce heat loss from the skin by abolishing sweating. Never cover the patient with a rubber sheet, and never overload him with blankets. If he feels hot to the touch do not hesitate to remove some of his coverings. The temperature in the theatre should be between 20–22°C, and the humidity about 60%.

(iv) Where it is obvious that the surgeon's manipulations are upsetting the patient, do not hesitate to ask that the patient be given a rest. A few minutes' pause without interference often gives the circulation a chance to recover, and thus prevents the onset of shock.

(v) The replacement of blood or fluid as necessary. This is discussed below.

Treatment of Shock on the Table

(i) Inform the surgeon.

(ii) Depress the head of the table to improve the cerebral circulation.

(iii) Administer a mixture rich in oxygen.

(iv) Administer intravenous fluids.

(v) There is increasing evidence that in shock, particularly of the endotoxic type, there is serious disturbance of the micro-circulation. This causes a loss of fluid into the tissues through increased permeability of the vessels. The administration of large doses of hydrocortisone intravenously, up to 1 g every hour, may be helpful.

Step (iv) requires amplification, conveniently approached by:

What are the anaesthetist's indications for an intravenous infusion?

(i) When shock has occurred, but preferably earlier.

(ii) In operations where shock or severe haemorrhage is likely to occur. Setting up the transfusion at the beginning of the operation saves untold trouble later in attempting rapidly to enter the collapsed veins of a shocked patient, who is also demanding your full attention at the head of the table. In addition, the use of a prophylactic transfusion lessens the possibility of the occurrence of shock. Do not insert the transfusion in the ward beforehand, for this not only disturbs the patient but the needle is likely to be pulled out on the way to the theatre.

(iii) Before operation in patients already shocked or grossly anaemic, or who are dehydrated.

(iv) It is better to set up an unnecessary transfusion than allow your patient to become dehydrated at any stage — during, before or after the operation. The advantage of an 'open' vein during any anaesthetic is a bonus.

Where is the best site to set up a transfusion?

(i) Never use the tempting antecubital veins except in emergency. There are usually satisfactory veins in the forearm and the back of the hand. The jugular veins should be reserved for emergencies.

(ii) It is best to insert the needle as far away from a joint as possible.

(iii) A drip should not be inserted into a leg vein, if a suitable arm vein is available. The risk of thrombosis, possibly complicated by embolism, is a real and serious sequel to transfusions in the leg.

(iv) If the patient is right-handed, it is a kindness to establish your drip in his left arm. This allows the patient to do much more for himself afterwards, and should he be so unfortunate as to develop a thrombosis his disability will be less.

How does one go about setting up a transfusion?

Make yourself used to a set routine that you will be able to follow in emergencies with exactitude and speed.

(i) Make sure you are in a comfortable position and have a good light on the arm; this cuts your difficulties in half. Select a vein and apply a thin rubber tourniquet above it. Place the tourniquet about three inches from the proposed site of puncture. Do not tie the tourniquet too tightly and so obstruct the arterial flow. Tie it with a knot you can release with one hand.

Aids in discovering and fully exposing a vein.
(a) Feel, not only observe, the patient's limb.
(b) Rub up the limb towards the tourniquet.
(c) Let the limb hang downwards for a short period.
(d) Warm the limb with hot-water bottles.
(e) Lightly flick or slap the vein you intend to use. This often has the effect of dilating it and making it more obvious.

The tourniquet should be applied as a first step, to allow the vein to become well distended.

(ii) Make up your mind whether to cut down or not. Simple puncture is preferable, as it is not invariably followed by thrombosis, the vein is available for further transfusions, the risk of sepsis is less, and insertion and removal of the needle are quicker and simpler. The use of a cannula instead of the standard needle allows a greater rate of flow, and having a "blunt" end is less likely to tear through the walls of the vein. Since blood and fluid may have to be replaced quickly and in large volumes, the largest possible cannula is better than two or more smaller cannulae or needles — and less confusing.

The procedure of cutting down is outlined below[1], the remainder of the technique of transfusion being the same.

(iii) Scrubbing up. Necessary when cutting down, no more necessary otherwise than when giving an intravenous injection. The outside of the transfusion set is not sterile, but you must avoid touching the needles.

(iv) Rapidly check your transfusion equipment. The essential requirements are:

(a) Sterile "giving" apparatus, of the plastic, disposable, type.

(b) Sterile swabs.

(c) Skin antiseptic (non-greasy and transparent).

(d) Drip stand.

(e) Four or five strips of strapping about 15 cm long.

(v) Remove plastic covers from piercing needle and air inlet. Insert piercing needle through the marked section in the transfusion bottle.

(vi) Clamp tubing below drip chamber. Hang up bottle and attach free end of air inlet to loop of bottle.

(vii) Squeeze and release filter chamber three or four times to fill with fluid. Release clamp to expel air from tubing and then tighten.

(viii) Clean skin over vein and insert needle.

(ix) Many infusion solutions are now prepared in plastic containers which collapse as they empty. Thus the remarks in (v) above do not apply. An air inlet is not necessary and the piercing needle will be introduced through a plastic seal on the container.

---

[1] For cutting down:

  (i) Scrub up.

  (ii) Thoroughly clean the site of operation.

  (iii) Make a small superficial horizontal incision over the vein.

  (iv) With blunt dissection, exposed 1–2 cm of the vein.

  (v) Push a Spencer Wells beneath the vein, returning it with the angle of a piece of thread bent double in its jaws.

  (vi) Divide the angle of the thread to make two separate pieces lying beneath the vein.

  (vii) Tie off the distal ligature.

  (viii) Nick the vein, steadying it with the proximal ligature.

  (ix) Insert the cannula, tying the proximal ligature round it.

Note.

(a) The vein may be steadied by a finger pressed alongside it, but beware of pressure sufficient to obliterate it.

(b) The skin should be pierced first at a point beside the vein, or behind the confluence of two veins.

(c) The needle is then moved slightly until it lies over the vein, in the line of the vein, and as nearly flush with the skin as possible.

(d) Pierce the vein gently, and equally gently run the needle about 2 cm up the lumen if possible. Success is proclaimed by a flow of blood, and failure often accompanied by a haematoma, to which you should apply a firm dressing before tackling a different vein.

(x) Release tourniquet and connect delivery tube after allowing a little fluid to flow from the end (avoidance of air embolism).

(xi) Whenever possible a cannula will be left in position rather than a needle. This must be strapped firmly to the skin with a narrow piece of adhesive tape passing below the cannula and crossing over in front "chevron-wise". This is to prevent loss of the plastic catheter should it fracture at the junction with the hub. Another piece of strapping will pass over the hub of the cannula. Form a loop of delivery tube immediately above the cannula, and strap the end of the loop nearest the bottle firmly to the limb, so that an inadvertent pull on the apparatus is not transmitted immediately to the needle. The remainder of the strapping may be applied according to choice, and may be augmented by a strip of 7·5 cm wide strapping to safeguard against movement of the cannula.

What fluids should be administered?

(i) If the patient's condition is due to loss of blood, then blood must be administered, the patient's own group being preferable to Group O blood. The blood of any patient undergoing major surgery should be grouped beforehand and each bottle should be cross-grouped. If cross-grouping has been performed before the operation, check the name on the prepared bottle with the patient's name on the operating list and on his notes before administering the blood. When massive transfusions are necessary, fluids (particularly blood, which is stored at 4°C) should be passed through a warming coil maintained at 40°C. If no special blood-warming apparatus is available, a plastic coil is inserted into the transfusion line and placed in a bucket of water kept at 40°C. If blood is pre-warmed, care must be taken to avoid excessive heating of the bottle, which might result in precipitation of protein (compare the boiling of an egg). It should be used as soon as possible, since decomposition will take place at normal temperature. Furthermore, blood once warmed cannot be returned to the blood bank for the use of another patient if not wanted, thus increasing the cost of the National Health Service and embarrassing the Government.

(ii) If the condition is not due to loss of blood, then:

(a) plasma (or, on occasions, serum)

(b) plasma substitutes (Dextran) or,

(c) normal saline, or

(d) 5% glucose in water (which has the advantage of not altering electrolyte balance by an excess of sodium ions)

may be injected. The plasma substitutes have the advantage that they are plentiful and are immune from the inherent danger in plasma of transmitting infective hepatitis. On the other hand, some of the plasma substitutes interfere with normal blood-grouping reactions. If the preparation is being given as an emergency measure, it is advisable first to take a sample of blood for grouping and cross-matching. Low molecular weight dextran (Dextran 40) deserves special mention because it reduces the viscosity of blood, and thus a tendency to sludge in cases where perfusion is impaired. Saline has a perfectly satisfactory though temporary action as it has no "water-holding" properties. Dextran 70 is frequently used as an alternative plasma substitute. Up to a litre may be given before its replacement by blood becomes essential (to avoid haemodilution).

How fast should the transfusion be run?

If blood is being lost in any quantity it must be replaced at the rate it is lost. This requires a certain amount of practice in its estimation. Remember that a fit adult can lose 0·5 litre of blood without great disturbance, but the loss of a further 500 ml will cause considerable deterioration in his condition. If blood has already been lost it should be replaced as soon as reasonably possible. The speed of the infusion may be hastened by compression of the fluid container (most are composed of soft plastic) or by a roller pump (Martin's) through which the drip tubing is led.

In shocked patients where there is no obvious bleeding to act as a guide the exact amount of fluid to be injected is often difficult to judge. It is sometimes forgotten that fractures cause haemorrhage into the tissues (up to a litre in the case of a fractured femur), and there can be loss into the abdomen or thorax after damage to viscera. In such cases a rapid transfusion should be started and continued until the condition of the patient improves. Haematocrit and haemoglobin estimations can be misleading, since haemoconcentration is the immediate response to blood loss, and is later followed by haemodilution. The circulating blood volume should give the answer we need, but direct measurement is difficult. Measurement of the central venous pressure provides a valuable guide, and should be performed in all cases where:

(a) Serious blood loss is expected.
(b) Extensive blood or fluid loss has already occurred and is being treated.

If this measurement is omitted, care must be taken against overloading the circulation, demonstrated by:

(a) Rising pulse with low blood pressure.
(b) Engorgement of veins, noticeable particularly in the jugulars, or a rise in the central venous pressure.
(c) Pulmonary oedema, first noticeable as crepitations at the lung bases.

The *central venous pressure* indicates the pressure of blood returning to the heart. To be scientifically accurate it should be taken in the right atrium. In practice, a catheter is usually introduced through the jugular, subclavian, or basilic veins and advanced until it reaches the superior vena cava. It may be connected to a simple water manometer, the base line of which is adjusted at the level of the right atrium — usually taken as the second sternal joint (the angle of Louis). The normal pressure is 4–10 cm of water, but it can be influenced by the efficiency of the heart and the respiratory pattern, apart from the circulating blood volume. Thus a central venous pressure measurement can be interpreted only in the light of other information, and is often more useful in indicating a trend in the pressure upwards or downwards.

What should be done if the drip stops?

Examine for and treat thus:

(i) Cannula moved slightly — gently rotate the limb and the needle.
(ii) Limb cold or a new bottle of cold fluid, sending the vein into spasm. Apply hot-water bottles to limb.
(iii) Tubing kinked.

(iv) Raising of operating table has diminished the head of pressure.

(v) Filter clogged (after several bottles of blood or plasma). The only remedy is to replace the giving set, which can be reconnected to the original cannula after first expelling air from the tubing.

(vi) Cannula clotted. If, there being no other obvious fault, positive pressure restarts the drip, then the vein is probably in spasm. If such pressure produces no result, then the cannula is probably clotted. If you believe this to be the case attach a syringe filled with saline solution and attempt to draw back blood. If none appears, inject the solution gently into the cannula. (The injection of a few ml of 1% procaine or 3–5 mg pethidine into the vein usually relieves the venous spasm promptly.)

(vii) Cannula out of the vein. Produces an ominous haematoma.

Careful examination of these points will go far to abolish the resigned attitude towards stopped drips, exemplified by one house-surgeon who maintained that intravenous transfusions were each of them possessed by the souls of fickle and perverse female devils.

Transfusion Reactions

It is to be hoped that after your scrupulous care in checking the patient's name, hospital number, blood group, and notes, the serial numbers on bottles, and cross matching (all of which should show a measure of agreement), you will never see the results of a mismatched transfusion. Should it occur, the products of the ensuing haemolysis will block and damage the kidneys to give rise to oliguria or even anuria. Hence early recognition may prevent too much of the wrong blood being given and minimise the damage.

The conscious patient will complain of headache, pain in the chest and in the loins, and feeling cold. He will probably be shivering, have rigors, be restless and short of breath, and exhibit all the signs of circulatory collapse. Under general anaesthesia this picture will be masked, but a reaction may be suspected if:

(i) There is an otherwise inexplicable hypotension.

(ii) There is a generalized capillary oozing from the wound.

In such circumstances, always check the transfusion bottle. Examination of the patient's blood will show haemolysis, and haemoglobin can be detected in the urine. Haemolytic jaundice will develop later.

In addition to the check carried out above, ensure also that the blood to be transfused has not been stored beyond its expiry date. Look also for any strange appearance of the blood. Haemolysis may occur from errors in storage, and may not always be easy to recognize. *Question any blood that looks doubtful in any way.*

Remember that blood is a potentially dangerous substance which can transmit disease, of which serum hepatitis is perhaps the most frightening. Australian antigen may be present in the blood of the patient, or in the blood to be administered. Contamination of the anaesthetist's hands at the time of venipuncture, or in setting up a transfusion, allows infection through breaks in the skin. Rubber gloves must always be worn in handling an affected patient, and strictly speaking whenever a blood transfusion is given.

Treatment

(1) Stop the transfusion and send the offending bottle, plus a further specimen of the patient's blood, to the laboratory.

(2) Give 500 ml of low molecular weight dextran by intravenous infusion.

(3) Put the patient on a careful fluid input and output chart.

(4) Restrict the fluid intake to match the total daily loss by bowels, sweat, urine (if any), etc. This will amount to about one litre.

(5) Give a high calorie (2,500 C) nitrogen-free diet.

(6) Ultimately, and if necessary, use haemodialysis with the artificial kidney.

Rectal Drip

A rectal drip, though not commonly employed, is still a useful and simple measure in the ward after operation. It is a means of modest fluid replacement if for any reason oral or intravenous routes cannot be used. Of the many solutions which may be given by this route, ordinary tap water is the cheapest and most satisfactory.

Heat Loss

Whenever there is fluid loss there is likely to be heat loss, because water lost by evaporation from a wound, sweat, or exhalation must be converted first into water vapour. This requires heat, which can be drawn only from the body. As administered fluids are often below body temperature and anaesthesia abolishes the normal heat-regulating mechanism, it is not surprising that many patients show a marked fall in body temperature. Because hypothermia depresses metabolism, the reactions to drugs may be abnormal and recovery from anaesthesia delayed. The use of a low-reading thermometer can be instructive and often surprising. Such inadvertent cooling is more likely to occur during long operations and where the incision is extensive, exposing large amounts of tissue. It is worse the more efficient the air conditioning in the theatre — particularly a theatre equipped with the recently introduced laminar flow. Here the air may be changed up to 400 times an hour.

Analeptics

Though the administration of intravenous fluids is the main treatment for shock, analeptics occasionally have their uses. Possibly their greatest help is in patients suffering from an overdose of drugs — particularly barbiturates. They are absolutely contraindicated in endotoxic shock.

In other forms of shock (particularly haemorrhagic) there is usually a cardiac element as well as failure of tissue oxygenation. It is therefore reasonable to administer small doses of analeptics to improve sympathetic activity and hence the contraction of the heart. A temporary improvement at least in blood pressure may be obtained, which is beneficial when there has been sudden hypotension, as may follow the administration of a spinal or extradural analgesic. There are many drugs on sale, of which metaraminol (Aramine) 2–3 mg and mephentermine (Mephine) 15 mg are popular. Mephentermine causes no overshoot of blood pressure nor rise in pulse rate. A more accurate control of the blood pressure can be effected with a nor-adrenaline (Laevophed) drip in a dilution of 1:250,000 or 1:500,000 in saline, but it should be used only by an expert.

Note that nikethamide and similar drugs are mainly respiratory stimulants, and are of most use in achieving at least a temporary improvement in a patient whose respiration has been depressed by centrally-acting drugs such as the barbiturates.

Arrhythmias

Cardiac arrhythmias may occur in patients suffering from pre-existing cardiac disease. Or, they may be provoked by anoxia, carbon dioxide excess, blood loss or reflex stimulation from manoeuvres carried out by the surgeon or anaesthetist. The significance of these induced cardiac irregularities may be difficult to assess, and their nature cannot be precisely diagnosed without the assistance of an ECG. A number of drugs are now available for the treatment of arrhythmias, but they must be used with considerable caution. Their unwise administration may have serious consequences, of which grave hypotension is perhaps the commonest. In unskilled hands the intravenous administration of 100 mg of lignocaine is probably safest, though propranolol (Inderal) and isoprenaline are more effective if properly used. Occasional irregularities unaccompanied by alarming signs are best ignored.

CHAPTER 9

Resuscitation

The Unconscious Patient

The commonest cause of unconsciousness in hospital practice is general anaesthesia, but the lessons learned from supervising anaesthetized patients can be applied equally well to cases of head injury, drug intoxication, neurological disease, or drowning. The problems are the same:

  (i) Avoidance of injury to the unconscious patient.

  (ii) Maintenance of efficient respiratory function.

Conditions like poliomyelitis, polyneuritis, and tetanus cause helplessness rather than unconsciousness, but when muscular control is extensively lost sufferers from these diseases may need to be treated in the same way.

Avoidance of injury. It is your duty to guard against injury from rings and watches, from pressures which might cause nerve palsies, from burns by hot bottles, electric blankets, heat lamps, and diathermy, and from falling out of bed. This list may be added to indefinitely, and as the results of these injuries may be both long lasting and difficult to treat, forethought and prevention are worth while.

Emergency artificial respiration. When breathing fails, urgent artificial respiration is required. Of the many means that have been advocated inflation of the lungs provides the most effective form of ventilation, and this can be achieved conveniently with mouth-to-mouth (or mouth-to-nose) respiration. The procedure may be lacking in aesthetic niceties, but it is effective and requires no apparatus. These two advantages cannot be questioned. The technique is as follows: the head is fully extended and the operator then pinches the subject's nose before applying his lips to those of the patient. On breathing out the operator should see the subject's chest expand. On removing his mouth the air should escape freely. This sequence

94

is repeated about 16 times a minute and continued as long as necessary. An airway must be maintained throughout, and to this end (and incidentally making it pleasanter for the operator) a Brook or a double ended airway may be used. Manual compression of the bag of an anaesthetic machine or resuscitator (Ambu bag, Oxford Inflating Bellows, etc.) may be performed instead.

Maintenance of efficient respiratory function. Efficient respiratory function can be maintained only through three closely related conditions:

(i) A clear airway.
(ii) A clear chest.
(iii) Adequate respiratory exchange.

All are dependent on each other, but of the three a clear airway is paramount in importance. To provide an airway it may be necessary to hold the jaw or tongue forward, to posture the patient for the same effect (tonsil position), to pass an oro- or naso-pharyngeal airway, to pass an endotracheal tube, or to perform a tracheostomy. The choice is determined by the circumstances, and often by the prognosis. All but tracheostomy must be considered temporary, though indispensable, forms of emergency treatment.

Where unconsciousness is expected to persist for a long time (weeks) an elective tracheostomy should be performed. This is a much safer procedure than one performed in a hurry later with inadequate lighting and no assistance.

Like tracheostomy, endotracheal intubation will provide

(a) a guaranteed airway, provided the endotracheal and tracheostomy tubes are cuffed to prevent secretions from the pharynx entering the respiratory tract
(b) a route for a suction catheter to the lower respiratory tract for the removal of secretions, etc.

The chest must be kept clear for gaseous exchange to take place efficiently. This means preventing the aspiration of vomit, pharyngeal secretions, blood, or other foreign matter, and the removal of any already there.

The methods available for this are:

(i) Emptying the stomach initially by the passage of a stomach tube — with suction handy in case of active vomiting during the process.
(ii) A gastric feeding tube, passed through the nose.
(iii) Postural drainage of the lungs, with changes of position every two hours.

(iv) Physiotherapy to encourage coughing.
(v) Aspiration of secretions by passing a suction catheter through the tracheostomy or endotracheal tube.
(vi) Bronchoscopy.

But more important than any of these is the patient's own ability to cough effectively.

Inadequate respiratory exchange from paralysis of the muscles of respiration requires artificial respiration. In many instances there is a choice between intermittent positive-pressure inflation, under manual control or by means of a specially designed pump, and an "iron-lung". Other methods are available, and have their uses. Although rigid rules cannot be given, the following guiding points may be helpful:

(1) The "iron lung" may occasionally be seen though very rarely nowadays, and is used where there is failure of respiration only.
(2) If respiration is adequate with respiratory obstruction, then posture (e.g., tonsil position) may be tried. If this fails, an endotracheal tube or tracheostomy must be employed. The commonest causes of failure with postural treatment are depression of consciousness, poor general condition (age or illness), and respiratory weakness with difficulty in coughing.
(3) Where there is both respiratory failure and obstruction to respiration the full treatment given above is required.

Note.

(1) Immediate post-operative respiratory failure can be treated with intubation and artificial respiration by squeezing the bag manually, or with a mechanical ventilator which is more reliable, predictable and efficient than you are.
(2) When treatment must be prolonged for six hours or more the air which ventilates the patient must be passed through a humidifier, or serious drying of the mucous membrane of the lower respiratory tract will make it impossible to remove secretions. Though preoccupied with the patient's respiration, you must not forget his general condition and must pay attention to hydration and feeding.

Finally, remember that unconscious patients die less from their primary lesions than from their chest complications. These are usually avoidable, but need the best treatment and nursing care available for their prevention. Antibiotics may be required to control secondary infection.

Tracheostomy

Though this procedure has figured prominently in the previous discussion, a few further words are needed. Tracheostomy has been promoted from a last hope for the dying to an essential part of the treatment in a variety of conditions not connected with unconscious patients. These include chest injuries, upper respiratory obstruction (tumours, infection, oedema, and paralysis of laryngeal nerves), and difficulties in swallowing without respiratory involvement (bulbar paralysis) to prevent food and secretions from soiling the trachea and lungs. In respiratory cripples it reduces their dead space and allows tracheobronchial toilet when coughing is ineffective.

The operation is relatively simple provided it is performed as an elective procedure and not in wild haste with a rusty penknife. Complications — which occur far more often in an emergency — include haemorrhage, pneumothorax, the operation performed too high or too low, wound infection, and associated injuries of the trachea and larynx. The tracheostomy tube may become blocked or dislodged and tracheal stenosis may develop as a late complication.

Special non-irritating plastic tubes passed through the nose may serve as an alternative and be left in place for 10–12 days.

Cerebral Oedema

Patients who suffer serious anoxic episodes, as might follow cardiac arrest or any of the conditions listed above, are liable to develop cerebral oedema. The signs are failure to regain consciousness, stertorous breathing, restlessness and twitching, raised temperature, and dilated pupils. Permanent damage may follow unless this is treated — by dehydration with 25% mannitol, or 30% urea, or 50% sucrose, or triple strength plasma. For rapid dehydration, frusemide (Lasix), 20 mg intravenously is worth while as an emergency measure. Hypothermia also can be used on occasions. If there is even a suspicion of cerebral oedema, do not wait for all the classical signs — do something.

In addition, it must be remembered that severe anoxia usually causes serious metabolic acidosis, which will require equally urgent treatment.

The Circulation

The ultimate aim of respiration is bringing oxygen to the tissues of the body and at the same time removing the product of cellular metabolism, carbon dioxide. Thus respiration itself is only the first stage of a wider process — the gases must still be transported between the lungs and the tissues. For this, the body depends on a sufficiency of haemoglobin as the carrying vehicle, and an efficient circulation promoted by the action of the heart.

Haemoglobin. The level of haemoglobin (normally about 15 g %) is usually considered a medical topic and cannot be discussed here in detail. But the anaesthetist must remember that patients anaemic from any cause will have a deficient oxygen-transport system, and need additional oxygen in the gases breathed. When the anaemia is due to acute blood loss, transfusion of whole blood will be needed to restore both the haemoglobin level and the circulating blood volume. If there is a risk of overloading the circulation the anaesthetist must give packed red cells, which do not affect the blood volume so much (roughly the same number of red cells for half the volume).

The Circulation. The circulating blood volume must be maintained by transfusion to correct losses from haemorrhage or dehydration (see p. 84). At the same time, the action of the heart must be maintained. This may be a suitable point to discuss the treatment of

Cardiac Arrest

occurring on the table, whatever the cause.
  (i) Inform the surgeon.
 (ii) Place the patient in the Trendelenburg position.
(iii) Give artificial respiration with oxygen, preferably through an endotracheal tube.
(iv) Perform cardiac massage without delay.

It has been shown that effective cardiac massage can be performed without opening the chest. With the patient lying on a firm surface,[1] the operator places one hand over the lower part of the sternum. His second hand is placed over the first. When he now leans forward his weight is transmitted to the patient's thoracic cage. The sternum is depressed and "squeezes" the heart against the vertebra. This compression should be carried out as rapidly as possible (about 60 times per minute) and must

---

[1] The manoeuvre is impossible to perform on a well sprung mattress, and the quickest way round the difficulty is to drag the patient on to the floor.

be vigorous, though undue enthusiasm has been known to fracture ribs, sternum, or vertebrae, and to rupture the liver. Even in such a situation, remember moderation in all things.

This procedure is clearly not limited to the operating room and can be applied equally well in the ward, the home, the street, or on the beach. On these occasions the operator will probably be single-handed. It then becomes necessary to divide attention between the cardiac and respiratory resuscitation. Perform about four squeezes of the chest and then interrupt the procedure to give one inflation of the lungs by the mouth-to-mouth method (see p. 94). The sequence may be repeated as long as necessary, but is exceedingly tiring for the operator. Help is therefore needed before your own efforts become ineffective.

The primary objectives are:

(a) Oxygenation of any blood which may be still circulating or can be made to circulate through the lungs.

(b) The establishment of a circulation through the coronary and cerebral vessels as soon as possible to avoid the permanent damage of prolonged anoxia.

If the heart stops — shown by no pulse, no blood pressure, and a disquieting pallor — no time must be lost in starting vigorous treatment. The brain tolerates three minutes of anoxia before incurring permanent damage. No apologies are offered in repeating some of the above advice, in the hope that the establishment of an emergency drill may save lives:

(1) Act immediately.

(2) Clear the airway.

(3) Establish artificial ventilation with oxygen and summon help.

(4) If pulseless, start external cardiac massage.

(5) Attach an electrocardiograph to determine whether the heart is in (a) asystole (b) ventricular fibrillation.

(6) Start an intravenous infusion and give 100–150 m.eq. of sodium bicarbonate.

(7) (a) If in asystole, administer 10 ml 1% calcium chloride, and if there is no response 10 ml 1/10,000 adrenalin directly into the heart.
(b) If in ventricular fibrillation, apply external electric defibrillation, which may be repeated if necessary.

(8) Continue external cardiac massage until the output is satisfactory.

(9) Continue artificial respiration.

(10) Consider (a) acid base balance (b) cerebral function.

CHAPTER 10

Post-operative Complications

The commonest post-operative complications are:
(1) Vomiting, sometimes complicated by dehydration.
(2) "Chests."
(3) Thrombosis of the leg veins, sometimes complicated by embolism.
(4) Carbon dioxide retention.
(5) Post-operative pain.
(6) Mechanical injuries.
(7) Delayed toxic effects of the anaesthetic drugs.

Post-operative Vomiting

Modern techniques have reduced the incidence of this sometimes distressing complication, but it would be foolish to claim that it never occurred. The vomiting reflex may be excited by so many stimuli, most of which are operative before, during, or after an anaesthetic, that the abolition of this sequel to an operation is most difficult. Consider the possible causes of post-operative vomiting and their prevention:

Before the anaesthetic

(i) *Personality of the patient.* Women and children (and indeed, cats and pigeons) vomit more easily than men. Fear and suggestion by example on the part of the other inmates of the ward are further potent causes of post-operative emesis. The nursing staff can do much in impressing the patients that vomiting is an exceptional sequel to modern anaesthesia and that they can look forward to a recovery period of complete tranquillity if they make up their minds to do so.

(ii) *Pre-operative morphine.* Morphine produces nausea in about 30 per cent of cases and induces vomiting in 10 per cent. Patients known to vomit readily after morphine and those in whom it is particularly desired to prevent vomiting (e.g., dia-

100

betics) may be given metoclopramide or some other specific antiemetic with morphine or pethidine premedication (see p. 15).

During the anaesthetic

(i) *The operation site.* Operations on the gut, on the gonads, and the mastoid region are examples of surgery of great vomiting potentiality.

(ii) *The anaesthetic agent.* Ether has been blamed, we consider far too enthusiastically, for the production of post-operative vomiting Cyclopropane is far from guiltless. Halothane and intravenous barbiturates have the reputation of causing least vomiting of all, but even their exclusive employment does not by any means abolish it. It occurs even after a simple nitrous-oxide anaesthetic, though in this case anoxia may well be to blame.

(iii) *Metabolic changes.* A patient undergoing an anaesthetic tends to become a diabetic, in that some degree of ketosis is likely to occur. The administration of fluids and glucose before operation may therefore be desirable.

(iv) *Irritation of the stomach.* Usual offenders:
    (a) Swallowed anaesthetic vapour.
    (b) Swallowed blood.
    (c) Hypoxia. Entirely your responsibility.

Post-operatively

(i) *Vomit bowls*, etc. Never allow a patient to recover consciousness in sight of an inviting vomit bowl, which receptacle must be placed behind the patient's head.

The vomiting rate in any ward usually varies directly with the force of the sister's personality. Patients must be told firmly that they must try not to be sick and that their recovery will not only be more pleasant but more rapid if the effort is made.

(ii) *Food and drink.* The regular use of light general anaesthesia (as opposed to deep general anaesthesia), and hence relatively complete recovery, allows a more liberal attitude towards fluid by mouth early during the post-operative period. Initially, an occasional sip of plain water may be permitted, and the use of a suitably flavoured mouthwash will go far to relieve the desire for a drink. Later, a small amount of fruit juice or even a cup of tea may be offered. The ingestion of large amounts of fluid may well produce vomiting, so it is advisable to test the patient's response to small quantities before returning to a normal diet. If the possibility of dehydration arises, the patient should be given an intravenous (or even a rectal) drip until drinking can be permitted.

(iii) *Morphine*. Remarks on this drug as premedication apply equally strongly after the operation. Pethidine is no substitute, itself liable to cause nausea and vomiting. An anti-emetic drug should be given also, if necessary.

(iv) *Causes other than post-operative*. The possibility of a cause unrelated to the operation must be borne in mind. We have seen a case of intestinal obstruction remain undiagnosed for two days after a plastic operation. The patient's surgical condition, e.g., cerebral tumour, may of course give rise to post-operative emesis.

(v) The modern passion for too early ambulation, before the effects of drugs have fully worn off.

Treatment

(a) If blood is being brought up from the stomach administer a dose of warm sodium bicarbonate solution, which will be returned, thus forming an effective stomach wash-out. This is followed by the treatment for cases without such complication:

(b) Stop all by mouth.

(c) Each year new drugs appear reputed to have powerful antiemetic properties, some related to the phenothiazine drugs. The one in most common use in your institution may be chosen with confidence (even if the confidence is only in the mind of the administrator). The three most commonly used at present are perphenazine in a dose of 2·5–5·0 mg, prochlorperazine 12·5 mg, or metoclopramide 5·0–10·0 mg.

(d) When the vomiting is persistent, say for more than 8 hours, dehydration is inevitable unless more active steps are taken. Treat with an intravenous infusion of 5% glucose in water. The degree of dehydration may be difficult to estimate clinically, in which case a continuous central venous pressure measurement should be taken (see p. 89) and fluids administered accordingly. Haemoglobin, haematocrit, electrolytes, urine analysis and other tests can be performed, but the delay before receiving the laboratory reports will reduce their usefulness.

Post-operative "Chests"

After operation the following chest complications may occur:

(i) Acute bronchitis, common and often pre-existing.

  (ii) Atelectasis, localized or more rarely massive. If untreated this may be complicated by infection.
 (iii) Bronchopneumonia — very common, particularly in the elderly. Often following, and confused with, the above.
 (iv) The results of acid regurgitation (see p. 105).
  (v) Lung abscess — usually due to inhalation of foreign bodies, including debris from septic teeth. This is a relatively late complication.

By far the most important of these conditions is localized atelectasis (often basal). The realization of this is highly important to the student who, possessing an even chance of developing into a house-surgeon, will then have to shoulder the entire responsibility of diagnosing and efficiently treating the condition.

Possible mechanism by which atelectasis is produced.
Early in the post-operative period, possibly even during the operation, plugs of mucus become lodged in some of the smaller bronchi. This leads to collapse of the lobule of lung behind the obstruction, which is then ripe for infection. Moreover, the cough power of the lobule is impaired so that voluntary removal of the obstruction is difficult. This sequence is, however, something of a hypothesis. Consider therefore:
Factors known by clinical observation to be associated with post-operative respiratory disease.
  (a) Operation site. Upper abdominals and hernias, particularly. All other operations are infrequently followed by such complications.
  (b) Sex. Predominantly male.
  (c) Smoking. Smokers are far more likely to suffer post-operative chest diseases.
  (d) Pre-existing respiratory disease. Chronic bronchitis is the usual offender. Except in emergency, never anaesthetize a patient suffering from a cold.
  (e) Heavy pre-operative and post-operative sedation, both of which allow the patient to sleep without moving for many hours after the operation. A badly given, deep general anaesthetic will have the same effect.
  (f) The unwise use of atropine, possibly, in that the drug produces a viscid mucus in the bronchial tree.
  (g) Disinclination of the patient to cough. This is particularly the case after the operations mentioned in (a), though it is probably not the entire explanation of the occurrence of "chests" in such cases.

(*h*) Position of the patient in bed after operation.
(*i*) Inhaled material.

Whatever form of anaesthesia is employed, and whatever general anaesthetic is chosen, the incidence of post-operative pulmonary disease remains substantially the same.

Diagnosis

Precluding any other obvious cause, any patient that:

(*a*) between 6 and 72 hours after operation
(*b*) shows a rise in temperature above 37°C
(*c*) has a sharp rise in pulse-rate
(*d*) particularly if accompanied by a disproportionate rise in respiration rate
(*e*) and particularly if a male recovering from an abdominal or hernia operation, is most likely suffering from a localized collapse of the lung. Alterations in temperature, pulse-rate and respiration rate often occur before there are any other clinical signs or symptoms. They may occur independently of each other, but should be regarded with suspicion and assumed to be atelactasis unless proved otherwise.

Later, depending on the extent of the area which is collapsed, the patient may appear ill and anxious: he may be dyspnoeic, and perhaps cyanosed. He is usually making unenthusiastic attempts to cough, with the production of little or no sputum.

Examination may reveal a shift of the mediastinum; there will most likely be dullness and diminished air entry at the base of one or both lungs. X-ray in the patient's bed will show opacities in the corresponding position, narrowing of the rib interspaces, and tracheal shift.

The picture given above is of a classical case of postoperative atelectasis. Remember, though, that few cases of any disease follow a textbook exactly. Atelectasis more than any other condition is one in which there is likely to be a striking disparity between the X-ray films, the clinical findings, and the appearance of the patient.

The diagnosis of massive lobar or pulmonary collapse, or of acute bronchitis, or of any other pulmonary condition, presents no more difficulty than in a medical ward. The treatment of these conditions is similarly well understood.

Treatment

(*a*) Removal of secretions. The patient must be made to

cough by tipping him over his bed with the affected side uppermost, holding his wound, heavily percussing his chest, and both encouraging him to cough and assuring him he will not burst open his wound in so doing. Breathing exercises, designed to expand the lungs, should preferably be carried out under the eye of a trained physiotherapist. This somewhat severe but effective treatment should ideally be repeated every two to three hours during the day, and though discretion must be used the most severely ill patients often require it the most. An expectorant mixture and inhalations may also be given, but neither can compare with the efficiency of the mechanical act of coughing.

If this treatment fails, suction through a bronchoscope passed under local analgesia may be required. Probably it is the coughing produced by the passage of the instrument and the subsequent manoeuvres that relieves the obstructed bronchi. If the previous treatment is effectively carried out, however, then the bronchoscopist should not appear in the ward. The longer the atelectasis persists, the more difficult is it to remove, and for this reason early recognition and vigorous treatment by the house-surgeon or ward sister is important. And the danger of the condition lies not only in adding another major illness to the patient's already enfeebled state, but in the possibility of later bronchiectatic changes in the ill-expanded lobules.

(b) Administer oxygen if necessary.
(c) If early resolution is not effected, prescribe the currently popular antibiotic or chemotherapeutic agent to prevent secondary infection.

Result of Acid Regurgitation

The inhalation of acid stomach contents is commonly seen in the obstetric department, where it has been given the title of Mendelson's syndrome. The condition undoubtedly can occur in other than obstetric cases, and is the effect of a small volume of acid material in the lungs — usually from an incompetent cardiac sphincter. The consequences are violent, frightening, and dangerous. The patient becomes dyspnoeic and cyanosed, the degree of bronchial spasm simulating a vicious asthmatic attack. Crepitations will be heard all over the chest, and pulmonary oedema may develop. An X-ray will show a generalized "snowstorm" appearance. Bronchoscopy is useless, other than as a means of making the patient cough, which is perhaps the most effective form of treatment. Coughing must be encouraged by any means at your disposal (see p. 102). Oxygen must be given and an antispasmodic such as aminophylline 250 mg with hydrocortisone 500 mg intravenously. In a serious case it will be necessary to establish an intravenous drip containing up to 1 g of hydrocortisone with 250 mg aminophylline in 500 ml of saline to produce a prolonged effect. The hydrocortisone may be more conveniently administered in equivalent doses of such preparations as dexamethasone. The more difficult cases — and indeed few are simple — may need in addition intermittent positive pressure ventilation, bronchial lavage, and cardiovascular support with digoxin, etc. Treatment is urgent and will tax the combined efforts of your consultants, so don't keep the problem to yourself.

Thrombosis and Embolism

Thrombosis in the deep veins of the legs is more common than was previously imagined, and, as with post-operative chest troubles, its aetiology is obscure but its active treatment must be enthusiastically pursued to forestall later disaster. The condition lies more under the care of the surgeon of the case than the anaesthetist, but the principles of treatment are important. Subcutaneous heparin in a dose of 5,000 units may be given six hourly, starting with premedication and continued for several days until the patient is ambulant. It has the disadvantage of causing unpleasant haematomata. Warfarin by mouth in a dose of 3–10 mg (depending on the prothrombin time) is becoming increasingly popular, but unfortunately must be continued for three to six weeks post-operatively. Anti-coagulants started before surgery will increase the bleeding, and the safety of such procedures must be monitored by daily prothrombin time estimations. The anaesthetist can assist in the prevention of thrombosis by seeing there is no pressure on the patient's calves during the operation and not interfering with the leg veins. To prevent venous stasis try crêpe bandages or elastic stockings. Better still, assist venous drainage by a slight head-down tilt throughout the operation.

There is little peace for the surgical patient these days. A distinguished anaesthetist we know, who was recently unfortunate enough to undergo an abdominal operation, recovered consciousness to discover a surgeon pinching his calves and a physician pummelling his chest crying "Cough!"

Carbon Dioxide Retention

Inadequate ventilation, most likely after a thoracic operation or in an emphysematous patient, steadily increases the carbon dioxide in the body. This has a narcotic affect and prolongs the anaesthetic. Indeed, prolonged unconsciousness or reversion to unconsciousness after temporary recovery may be its most obvious feature. Cyanosis develops only when the respiratory centre has been poisoned with carbon dioxide. In this event the pulse is found to be slow and bounding, with a raised blood pressure. Circulatory collapse occurs later.

Although the condition is primarily due to inadequate ventilation, it may be aggravated by anaesthetic drugs. Treatment is by efficient artificial respiration (intubation, followed by inflation of the lungs with air or oxygen) to "wash out" the carbon dioxide. It may be necessary to continue this for two hours or more to allow time for the respiratory centre to recover. Analeptics and other such drugs are a waste of your time and the taxpayers' money.

Post-operative Pain

Pain is not an inevitable sequel to surgery, but it is a significant complication in well over half the patients. Those likely to suffer most will have undergone thoracotomy, upper abdominal operations, or haemorrhoidectomy, but pain is an individual problem which is not always related to the severity or site of an operation. Treatment is important, for unrelieved pain can cause hypotension and inadequate ventilation, quite apart from the mental and physical distress.

Pethidine, morphine, and papaveretum are the three drugs most commonly employed systemically, but all can cause respiratory depression and hypotension if used unwisely. It is all too often overlooked that a man who enters the operating theatre as an A1 life can come out in medical category C3. The dose of a drug which was suitable before will now be a gross overdose, as the result of blood loss, trauma, and general anaesthesia. It is usually better to order a small dose which can be repeated if necessary rather than too much to start with. In any case, it should be less than the dose ordered for premedication.

Do not forget the simple analgesics such as aspirin and codeine. Both can give considerable relief, particularly in cases where the pain is not severe enough to warrant more powerful drugs.

Alternatively, some form of continuous local analgesic block — usually extradural — may be employed (see p. 121). The technique necessitates the introduction of a fine catheter, preferably at the mid-point of the nerve segments involved. By so doing, an effective block can be produced with a volume of local analgesic solution sufficiently small (often no more than 5·0 ml) that it will not spread and cause extensive motor paralysis or hypotension. The use of lignocaine requires "topping up" doses every two hours or so, but bupivacaine (Marcain) is often effective for six hours or more, simplifying management. Thoracic extradurals are of particular value for the relief of pain after thoracotomy and upper abdominal operations. Caudals can be a source of great comfort after haemorrhoidectomy, and ideally should be continued until after the first bowel movement.

Bupivacaine has considerably extended the use of local analgesia by single injection technique. Thus intercostal or axillary block can start the patient after an operation with freedom of pain for several hours. Fear of pain is very real, and even a few pain-free hours of recovery are invaluable.

Remember that the total abolition of pain makes a patient intolerant of even minor discomfort when the block wears off, and with lack of normal sensations the full bladder or rectum may be overlooked.

All this requires careful supervision and attention to asepsis, and is therefore suitable only in selected cases and in experienced hands.

Mechanical Injuries

These occur not only in the post-operative period but during the whole time that the patient is unconscious and unable to take care of himself. They include such disasters as postural nerve palsies, burns from hot surfaces, physical injury resulting from falling off the trolley or careless lifting of the stretcher, etc. They can be prevented only by watchfulness and forethought.

Delayed Toxic Effects

Foremost in the anaesthetist's mind at present are hepatitis after the administration of halothane (see p. 50) and renal damage following methoxyflurane (see p. 58). The consequences of these and other vapours on theatre personnel must also be borne in mind (see p. 59). When these drugs are used, others which may harm the liver (e.g., barbiturates) or kidneys (e.g., streptomycin) must be eschewed. When liver and renal function is reduced, the choice of halogenated anaesthetic agents must be made warily. There is evidence that a previous anaesthetic with one agent may predispose to more serious consequences from another.

CHAPTER 11

Local And Spinal Analgesia

The Most Important Factor in Local and Spinal Analgesia

Be perfectly certain you are injecting the correct drug.

Drugs

Although there are many local analgesics manufactured (and advertised), the following are the most commonly used:

(1) Lignocaine (Xylocaine).
(2) Prilocaine (Citanest).

Not forgetting:

(3) Procaine (Novocaine) the original synthetic preparation, the cheapest and still of use.
(4) Cocaine, the only one to produce vasoconstriction and the most toxic.
(5) Bupivacaine (Marcain), a recent addition.
(6) Cinchocaine (Nupercaine), still used for spinal analgesia.

The properties of these different drugs can be conveniently listed in tabular form:

	Maximum Dose*	Concentration	Duration	Main Uses
Lignocaine	500 mg	0·5–2%	90 mins	Topical, nerve block, extradurals.
Prilocaine	600 mg	0·5–2%	90 mins	Topical, nerve block, extradurals, i.v. regional.
Procaine	1,000 mg	0·5–2%	60 mins†	Nerve block, infiltration.
Cocaine	150 mg	1·0–4%	20 mins	Topical.
Bupivacaine	150 mg	0·5%	300 mins+	Extradural, nerve block.
Cinchocaine	150 mg	0·02%	120 mins	Spinals.

* There are always fools about who are prepared to ignore the maximum safe dose of any drug. Ignorance in law is not a valid excuse — neither is it in medicine.

† With adrenalin.

110

Adrenalin. With the exception of cocaine all local analgesic drugs cause vasodilatation. To counteract this effect, and thus slow the rate of absorption of the drug into the blood stream, adrenalin is usually added to most local analgesic solutions. The result is twofold:

(a) The drug remains at the site of injection longer, which prolongs the analgesia.

(b) The chances of a toxic dose reaching the circulation are much reduced.

Adrenalin should never be used in a concentration stronger than 1/200,000, but can be effective in a solution as weak as 1/600,000. The total dose should never exceed 0·5 ml of a 1/1,000 solution (0·5 mg).

The technique of local analgesia may be considered under the headings:

(1) Surface analgesia.
(2) Infiltration of tissues.
(3) Nerve block.
(4) Field block.
(5) Intravenous regional analgesia (for the limbs).

(1) Surface analgesia.

(i) *Drugs.*

(a) Cocaine, 1–4%.

(b) Lignocaine or prilocaine, 4%. This is the only occasion on which this high concentration is used.

The agent may be used in a spray, applied as an ointment or cream, or painted on the mucous membrane directly. A lozenge of amethocaine (60 mg) may be sucked before laryngoscopy or bronchoscopy.

(ii) *Uses.*

(a) Minor surgery of the eye

(b) laryngoscopy and bronchoscopy

(c) incision of quinsy (never give a general for this)

(d) S.M.R. and nasal polypectomy

(e) cystoscopy

are a few of the procedures possible under this form of local analgesia.

(2) Infiltration Analgesia.

(i) *Drugs.* Lignocaine or prilocaine, 0·25–0·5% are the drugs most commonly used. Adrenalin is usually added to the solution.

(ii) *Uses.* Any minor surgery where sepsis is not present and the patient can be guaranteed to co-operate (as a rule, children are unsuited for local analgesia). The drug is injected fanwise through as few needle pricks as possible. If the point of the needle is kept moving as the fluid is ejected the possibility of inadvertent intravenous injection is minimized, the advancing stream of fluid pushing away small blood vessels. The technique is simple, requires no anatomical knowledge and is effective. Extraction of single teeth, except mandibular molars, may be accomplished after a little 2% solution has been infiltrated into the surrounding gum. The needle is inserted into the deepest point in the adjoining buccal sulcus, towards the apex of the tooth, and the injection repeated on the palatal aspect.

In addition, infiltration analgesia may be combined with general anaesthesia, or major nerve blocks, often with the aim of providing a bloodless field by making use of the vasoconstrictor effect of the adrenalin in the solution.

(3) **Nerve block (conduction analgesia).**

This technique requires greater accuracy than the foregoing, for the nerves concerned must be located exactly. The secret of success lies in a knowledge of anatomy which allows specific nerves to be related to good landmarks, preferably bony.

(i) *Drugs*. Lignocaine and prilocaine have become the usual choices in a 1–2% solution.

(ii) *Uses*. Some of the commoner nerve blocks are:

(a) Block of the inferior dental and lingual nerves in the region of the mandibular foramen, for extraction of the molar teeth.

(b) Brachial block, originally performed above the clavicle just lateral to the subclavian artery. Since there is risk of causing a pneumothorax, an axillary approach, which achieves the same effect, is now more widely used. This nerve block allows any operation to be performed upon the arm below the elbow.

(c) Finger block, for operation upon the finger where general anaesthesia is not employed. The solution is infiltrated round the base of the finger to affect the digital nerves. This is a satisfactory technique, but—

(i) always avoid adrenalin in the analgesic solution,

(ii) always avoid a tourniquet round the finger,

both to prevent possible post-operative gangrene.

(d) Intercostal nerves, reached below their respective ribs for the relief of pain (e.g., fractured ribs), but there is a risk of damaging the underlying pleura and lungs, causing a pneumothorax.

(4) **Field block** is of use where the anatomy of the operation permits it. A barrage of local analgesic solution is laid across the path of the nerves supplying the operation field e.g. the scalp.

(5) **Intravenous drugs** may be injected for local analgesia of the limbs.

This technique has been revived recently and is of particular value in the out-patient. An indwelling needle is inserted in a vein on the dorsum of the hand or foot, the limb is exsanguinated and a tourniquet applied before injection. Prilocaine 0·5% is used in volumes of about 40 ml for an arm and 80 ml for a leg. Analgesia develops rapidly and passes off equally quickly when the tourniquet is removed (not earlier than 15 minutes after injection for fear of toxic reactions). The method works excellently in the arm but is more difficult to apply and potentially more dangerous in the leg because of the greater volume of drug needed.

Indications for Local Analgesia

The indications for local analgesia are, briefly:

(a) minor surgery,

(b) where the life of the patient may be endangered by his being made unconscious,

(c) unskilled anaesthetist,

(d) the nature of the operation (e.g., drainage of empyaema, bleeding in upper air passages),

(e) lack of skilled nursing,

(f) a recent meal,

(g) diagnostic and therapeutic procedures,

(h) patients who may be conveniently so operated upon and present some lesion making a general anaesthetic undesirable (e.g., a tendon repair in the forearm when active movement by the patient may assist the surgeon by identifying the structures).

The contra-indications are:

(a) sepsis near the field of injection,

(b) non-co-operation by the patient.

(c) major surgery in which, to be effective, so much local analgesic solution would have to be injected that there would be risk of a toxic reaction.

Premedication for patients undergoing an operation under local analgesia should be heavier than for general anaesthesia.

Dangers

Whenever an injection is made there is a risk that neighbouring structures may be damaged by the needle point. Thus, the thoracic and abdominal contents are especially susceptible to injury, such as,

(i) pneumothorax (tension pneumothorax if the substance of the lung is torn)

(ii) infection of needle track after puncture of bladder or gut

(iii) serious haemorrhage from injury to the spleen, especially if it is enlarged by disease.

Always remember that a distended abdomen has a very thin wall.

Apart from trauma, injection or application of a local analgesic may be followed by rapid collapse and possibly death due to the following causes:

(1) **Overdose.** It is equally important to avoid administering an overdose of "local" as of a general anaesthetic. The maximum safe doses listed earlier in this chapter refer to fit, healthy adults. They must be considerably reduced in "the young, the old, and the ill".

What matters is the total dose administered and the site of injection — a relatively small amount in a highly vascular area is more dangerous than a larger dose where the blood supply is limited.

An overdose occurs when the rate of absorption (or of administration in case of an inadvertent intravenous injection) exceeds the rate at which the body can destroy or neutralize the drug. This rule applies to any drug. In the case of a local analgesic, a toxic reaction is characterized by bradycardia, restlessness, and convulsions. The convulsions indicate cerebral irritation and are indistinguishable from other types of convulsions (e.g., eclampsia, epilepsy), Bradycardia signifies depression of the myocardium and blocking of the conducting mechanism of the heart. The treatment is:

1. Stop the administration.
2. Check the patient's airway.
3. Give oxygen.
4. Perform artificial respiration if necessary.
5. Control convulsions by the intravenous injection of a minimal quantity of thiopentone. As this will also depress the heart, it may be better, if you are competent to pass an endotracheal tube, to inject suxemethonium to control the fit.

6. If the overdose has been sufficient to produce cardiac arrest, treat this condition as described on page 98.

Occasionally, the reaction ascribed to a local analgesic solution is, in fact, due to the adrenalin it contains. Such a reaction can be distinguished from an overdose of a local analgesic by the pallor of the patient, and the rapid, almost impalpable, pulse. There may be cardiac irregularities and a brief but dangerous rise in blood pressure. If the patient is conscious he will be anxious and complain of headache, nausea, and palpitations. The systemic effect of adrenalin is transient, and although there is no specific treatment for such a reaction, recovery, if it is to take place, will be spontaneous. Unfortunately, many cases end in ventricular fibrillation, needing electrical defibrillation and full scale cardiac resuscitation if there is to be any hope of survival.

(2) **Inadvertent intravenous injection.** Always draw back the syringe plunger when injecting more than 2 ml of local analgesic at one point.

(3) **Idiosyncrasy.** Sudden collapse immediately following injection of small quantities of local analgesic is a disquieting phenomenon, but is so rare that it is doubtful whether it is a true idiosyncrasy. In many instances, it is undoubtedly due to an inadvertent intravenous injection of the drug.

(4) **General.** Large-scale blocks (spinal, extradural, etc.) can cause a serious fall in blood pressure and paralyse the intercostal muscles to such an extent that respiration becomes embarrassed. Such effects must be constantly guarded against, and treated thus:

(i) Tilt down the head of the table.
(ii) Give oxygen.
(iii) Start a transfusion.
(iv) Give a vasopressor agent. Metaraminol, in a dose of 2–3 mg, is good and is found in most hospitals.

Spinal Analgesia

The indications for spinal analgesia are mainly a matter of opinion. These opinions have to some extent been formed by medicolegal decisions, but happily more rational and strictly medical reasons are returning to favour. ''Spinals'' are a disagreeable form of analgesia to many patients, and are potentially dangerous unless employed with great care and attention. They are certainly not to be regarded as simple substitutes for experience and skill in general anaesthesia.

As a general rule, spinal analgesia should not be used for:

(1) Children.
(2) Ill and feeble patients.
(3) Patients with an unsound cardiovascular system.
(4) Patients with severe abdominal distension — unless you are competent to deal with the inadequate respiration which follows paralysis of the intercostal muscles when the diaphragm is already "splinted".
(5) Patients with central nervous diseases such as tabes, disseminated sclerosis, or syringomyelia — you will certainly be blamed for any exacerbations, although it is doubtful whether the spinal analgesic is concerned in any way at all.

Advantages

An advantage of a spinal analgesic, apart from the provision of profound relaxation without need for a reasonably skilful general anaesthetic, is the retention of consciousness by the patient. A second is the non-irritation of the lungs by the agent — an attribute with no influence on the post-operative "chest" rate whatsoever. A further distinction in the eyes of some is lack of haemorrhage at the time of operation. This is effected by an overall fall in blood pressure, which carries its own particular risks; and there is always the possibility that bleeding may occur when the blood pressure rises again after the patient has returned to bed.

Disadvantages

The disadvantages of "spinals" are:

(1) A large fall of blood pressure, usually related to the level of the spinal block. It is probably due to a paralysis of the sympathetic nervous system when the level reaches the 10th thoracic segment or above. In addition, the adrenals will be virtually denervated.
(2) Possible interference with efficient respiratory exchange.
(3) Possible technical difficulties in administration by the inexpert.
(4) Post-operative vomiting and chest complications are just as common as after general anaesthesia.
(5) The relatively high incidence of post-operative headaches.

Particular dangers
(1) Meningitis, due to failure on the part of the anaesthetist to guarantee absolute sterility for his equipment or for his technique of using it.
(2) Post-operative neurological sequelae, e.g., cauda equina lesions, cranial nerve palsies, myelitis, etc.
(3) Respiratory or circulatory failure, already mentioned under the disadvantages.

Technique of Spinal Analgesia

The watchword is "complete and certain sterility in administration". All equipment and ampoules of local analgesic drugs must be sterilized by autoclaving.

Apparatus. The essentials are:
   (i) Spinal needle and stilette.
  (ii) Syringe for spinal analgesic.
 (iii) Large-bore needle for drawing up spinal analgesic.
  (iv) A separate syringe and hypodermic needle for local infiltration to the skin.
   (v) A file for local analgesic ampoules.
  (vi) Ampoules of the local analgesic solution to be injected into the sub-arachnoid space.
 (vii) A coarse needle for puncturing the skin of the back before inserting the spinal needle.
(viii) Swabs.
  (ix) Swab holder.
   (x) Sterile towels.

All these should be prepared and autoclaved together on a special tray. Each tray should contain one set only. In addition:
  (xi) An effective skin antiseptic such as 0·5 per cent chlorhexidine (Hibitane) must be available.

Technique of injection.
This may be performed with the patient sitting or lying on the trolley. In both cases request "the chin to touch the knees" in order to open the intravertebral spaces as much as possible and so facilitate the task.

After donning a cap and mask the anaesthetist must scrub up thoroughly and pull on sterile rubber gloves. He should then prepare his apparatus and draw up the solution to be injected into the theca in the syringe put aside for this purpose. The remainder of the "spinal" solution may be drawn up in the skin-wheal syringe.

A wide area of the patient's back should now be carefully cleaned. The swabs must be held in the swab holder to avoid contaminating the gloves. A sterile towel is now draped around the bottom of the back (or lower loin) and the site of puncture selected. This is most safely performed between the third and fourth lumbar vertebrae, as the cord occasionally ends below the generally accepted level of L 1-2. The space may be found by feeling the two iliac crests through the sterile towel, as the inter-vertebral level L 3-4 lies at the same level. Inject a small bleb of local solution subcutaneously: this is your "target". Puncture the skin with the coarse needle, and pass the spinal needle through the hole it has made. The spinal needle must be held only by the hub, and inserted into the tissues exactly in the midline and in a slightly upward direction. If it is necessary to touch the shaft of the needle to facilitate its smooth insertion, do so through a sterile gauze swab.

The needle may:

(i) Pierce the dura with a slight but distinct sudden loss of resistance. Removal of the stilette is followed by a flow of C.S.F., proclaiming success.

(ii) Meet with complete resistance. This means that bone has been encountered, and the needle must be withdrawn to the skin, changed in direction slightly, and a second attempt made. If three attempts fail, choose the space higher or lower. If three endeavours in the alternate space are unsuccessful it is advisable to abandon the project, for more attempts are likely to be followed by sepsis.

(iii) Emit blood. Withdraw to the skin and try again.

Up to now you have followed the course to be taken whenever a lumbar puncture is made, and it is therefore hoped that this description will be of value to you in the wards even if you never give a spinal analgesic in your life.

Once the dura has been pierced, attach the syringe to the needle and inject the analgesic. A little C.S.F. may be withdrawn into the syringe to give assurance of a free flow, but if this is repeated too many times the local analgesic solution may become sufficiently mixed with the C.S.F. to produce an uncontrolled high spinal.

The basic steps so far described are applicable to all types of spinal analgesic not demanding a technique suitable only for experts. The treatment of the patient thenceforward differs according to the type of spinal analgesic used.

The only technique to be considered by the student is:

Heavy Spinal Analgesia

C.S.F. has an almost constant specific gravity in the region of 1·004. It is therefore obvious that a solution with a higher specific gravity will fall, and a solution with a lower specific gravity will rise, in the dural sac of a patient in the upright position.

This must be remembered when a "head down" position is required to combat the effect of a fall of blood pressure or to satisfy a gynaecologist. In addition, the natural curves of the spine have a limiting effect. T 6 is the lowest point in the thoracic curve of a patient lying on his back, and since a heavy solution cannot run uphill it is most unlikely that the analgesic level can rise above T 4.

The heavy solution. In the U.K., cinchocaine 1/200 with glucose added, giving a specific gravity of 1:025 (C.S.F. 1:004), has been the most usual agent. There has been difficulty in obtaining this preparation, and it is possible that mepivacaine (Carbocain — which has a rather brief duration) will become the agent of choice. It is used in exactly the same way as cinchocaine, and comments about one may be applied equally to the other. The onset of analgesia with cinchocaine occurs in about fifteen minutes. Both will last for about two hours. The drugs are "fixed" in about 10–15 minutes after injection, when further movements of the patient will not alter the level of analgesia.

Dosage scheme.

Operation Site			Dose	Position of Patient
Perineum	...	...	0·5 ml	Sitting
Lower abdomen up to				
umbilicus	...	...	1·5 ml	Lateral
Upper abdomen		...	2·0 ml	Lateral with 5° Trendelenburg tilt

Care of the Patient Under Spinal Analgesia

(1) Pre-operatively

The same preparation is required as for a general anaesthetic, except that the premedication may be heavier, especially if the patient is to remain conscious.

(2) During the operation

These remarks apply equally well to operations performed under local analgesia.

   (i) See the patient is comfortable on the table.

  (ii) Someone must pass the entire operation at his head, observing blood pressure and adequacy of respiration and affording him encouragement and diversion.

 (iii) The surgeon must not be permitted to describe his progress in audible tones, nor to employ his patient's chest as an instrument tray.

 (iv) For every spinal analgesia which involves the abdominal wall it is advisable to administer oxygen.

  (v) Faintness and nausea may accompany moderate falls in blood pressure and are particularly noticeable during surgical manipulations in the upper abdomen. These complaints must be treated on their own merits, and while sips of water and cold sponging of the patient's face may be helpful in mild cases, more active steps are needed if the faintness results from a serious fall in blood pressure.

 (vi) It is not unreasonable to sedate any patient who might otherwise remain widely awake during the course of an operation under any form of local analgesia. If there is no contraindication, diazepam intravenously in a dose of 5–10 mg is efficient and will allay restlessness. In extreme cases, a small dose of thiopentone followed by nitrous oxide and oxygen can be used.

(3) Post-operatively

Post-operative treatment raises two important points:

   (i) Avoidance of injury (especially thermal) to limbs still insensitive to pain.

  (ii) Prevention of post-operative headache. The patient should lie with the foot of the bed raised and in semi-darkness for the first six hours after operation. Reading and smoking should be prohibited for a further six hours. Treatment of such headache is difficult, but since it is aggravated by raising the head it is obvious that a supine or prone position is essential. The administration of codeine or pethidine is helpful and the patient should be encouraged to drink as much as possible.

Extradural Block

The extradural space extends from the base of the skull to the sacral hiatus. It lies within the vertebral canal, separating the dura mater and its contents from the bony vertebral wall. It is traversed by the spinal nerves, which leave the canal via the intervertebral foramina, to be distributed to their various dermatomes. Local analgesic solution in the extradural space will thus affect these nerves *outside* the dural sheath. By preserving the integrity of the dura mater, headaches and the neurological complications which may follow spinal analgesia are avoided. Otherwise the results are similar, though rather less predictable, as solution "leaking out" through the intervertebral foramina prevents accurate assessment of how far a given volume will spread.

Technique. The extradural space may be reached at any level. The technique is similar to that of an intrathecal injection, but the needle having penetrated the ligamentum flavum stops short of the dura mater. A larger volume of solution (1·5% lignocaine) must be used. In the thoracic region, the procedure is modified by inserting the needle 1 cm lateral to the spines and aiming medially and upwards to reach the ligamentum flavum in the mid-line — thus overcoming the obliquity of the spines. Knowing that your needle is in the extradural space requires some skill and experience.

Their advantages over spinals allow extradural blocks to be used for a variety of therapeutic as well as surgical reasons. These include the control of pain in labour, and the management of post-operative pain and of pain arising from fractured ribs (for which a limited segmental block by the thoracic approach is recommended). But they are not foolproof — a fall in blood pressure, paralysis of the respiratory muscles, inadvertent spinal injection, toxic reactions to the analgesic, and a rather more difficult technique suggest that they should not be undertaken too lightly.

Caudal analgesia. This is a form of analgesia in which the extradural space is reached through the sacral hiatus. The technique is rather easier than the lumbar approach and — there being little danger of piercing the dura mater — certainly safer. The hiatus lies between the two cornua of the sacrum and is identified by direct palpation. This form of analgesia is particularly useful when the sacral nerves only are the primary target — cystoscopy, haemorrhoidectomy, and of course during labour.

CHAPTER 12

The Choice of Anaesthetic

Although there can be no hard and fast rule governing the choice of anaesthetic, and all the possible contingencies cannot be discussed, this chapter is intended to guide the student in deciding what anaesthetic to administer — a decision that must be clearly made before the induction is started.

The problem is not as difficult as it first appears. In fact, there are probably not more than two possible choices, even though the larger textbooks might suggest that there is · a specific anaesthetic agent and technique for every operation. You can make your decision by answering the question "What anaesthetic am I most competent to administer?"; or if you prefer it "What anaesthetic in my hands is likely to be safest for the patient?" If you are honest — and in this case dishonesty might lead to the death of the patient — your choice will probably lie between the combination of nitrous oxide, oxygen, and halothane or ether, or open ether in unsophisticated surroundings. In many instances, small refinements may be added — e.g., a "sleep" dose of thiopentone to make the induction pleasanter, or trichlorethylene or halothane to facilitate the introduction of ether.

Do not try to emulate the specialist. He has learned from years of experience and the sharp realization of his own limitations. So be ready to acknowledge yours, and don't be talked into doing something beyond your capabilities. Misplaced enthusiasm and the belief that methods recommended by some book or other are the best, though you have never practised them, lead to accidents. Remember that the most important person in the operating theatre is the patient, and his safety is of primary importance.

The methods that we recommend are not necessarily the best, but we believe that they are safe, and less likely to get you into serious trouble than many others.

Considerations concerning the Patient

(1) *Children.* Give pre-operative medication as described on pages 14 & 16. Ether is excellent for children but introduction of this irritant vapour may be eased by first giving small quantities of halothane. Induction with nitrous oxide is best performed by running the gas under cover of the head blanket towards the face of a child already asleep under the effect of premedication. This technique calls for the most gentle transference of the patient from bed to theatre, and an absence of any interference to his sleeping position once arrived. Sisters must be firmly discouraged from pulling back the covers and sitting up the child "to see the funny man" on arrival in the anaesthetic room. Talking and other noise should be similarly condemned. With slight modifications this can be applied to the conscious child as well. The child's attention must be held during the induction by suitable conversation — we have found favourite foodstuffs or pets topics likely to maintain interest even under such adverse conditions. Once the respiration becomes regular, apply the face-piece and continue the induction. Non-co-operative children can rarely be deceived into "blowing up the football", "smelling the scent", and so forth, so that patience and tact in securing the confidence and co-operation of youngsters are well rewarded.[1]

Alternatively, ether on an open mask may be given after induction with halothane (which can be administered by drop also, but slowly and with more caution) but the smell in high concentration can be unpleasant. It is therefore all the more necessary to exercise extreme care when you try to induce a small child. As soon as consciousness is lost, the mask is placed on the face and you change to ether as soon as possible. You must never persist with halothane in an attempt to produce deep anaesthesia, since it will present difficulties which are better overcome by a more highly paid servant of the State.

The ether should be "dropped" over all the surface of the mask as a steady stream of drops rather than in intermittent

---

[1] The advantage of adequate premedication for children is illustrated by the true story of a distinguished London surgeon and his anaesthetist who arrived, one hot summer morning, at the country seat of one of our noblemen. Their mission was the removal of tonsils and adenoids from the young heir to the title. The operation was to be staged in a drawing room, from which french windows led on to a historic lawn. No sedative having been administered, on arrival in the theatre the patient promptly took fright and bolted for it through the open windows, his medical advisers in heavy pursuit. After he had led them a wonderful dance in the shrubbery they finally got him in a hot-house.

douches. Give ether as fast as the patient will tolerate it — nothing is gained by deepening anaesthesia slowly. When it is obvious that a reasonable concentration of ether is causing no disturbance in respiration, it may be increased still further by placing a piece of Gamgee tissue between the face and the mask. This enables a tight fit to be maintained, reducing the dilution of ether vapour with air.

During an open administration note:

(i) A perfect airway is essential.

(ii) While "talking" your patient to sleep, a large quantity of your induction agent may be put on the mask: when the mask is lowered, a dangerous amount may still be present.

(iii) Ether cannot be vaporized easily from a mask that has frozen: always have a spare mask handy.

(iv) When the mask is wet with ether and condensed exhalations it becomes relatively impermeable to gases and there may be an appreciable build-up of carbon dioxide. Change the mask.

(2) *Old and ill* persons will be found to require little of any anaesthetic, general or local, but they must be treated with great care. Be guarded in the use of thiopentone and ensure adequate oxygenation.

(3) Patients with respiratory disease, e.g., bronchitis or tuberculosis, are best given a non-irritant vapour. A low spinal may be administered for suitable operations. Never anaesthetize any case with active respiratory disease, which includes the cold, unless strictly necessary.

(4) *Cardiac disease* demands considerable care for full oxygenation. As a rule, however, most persons with cardiac lesions stand anaesthesia extremely well unless they are in failure. Because of the obvious danger of hypotension producing a deficient coronary circulation and interference with respiratory function, it is inadvisable to administer a spinal analgesic to any patient with severe cardiac disease unless the analgesia can be limited to the sacral nerves.

(5) *Diabetic patients* who are well controlled require no special preparation for elective surgery, and their régime should be disturbed as little as possible. If this is based on long-acting insulin, conversion to treatment with soluble insulin is essential, except in fit, well stabilized patients who are undergoing minor elective operations. The dose of soluble insulin should be related to blood sugar estimations, but a crude guide is to give approximately half the lente insulin dose as soluble units

and repeat this some eight hours later. If the patient is unable to take food by mouth, this must be compensated by a glucose infusion. But serious attention must be paid to the patient who is found to be diabetic immediately before an emergency operation, or the known diabetic out of control (most commonly as a result of infection). In such cases, the correction of dehydration, electrolyte balance, and infection are important. It is better for the patient to arrive in the theatre hyperglycaemic, provided there is no ketosis, than to risk the serious results of hypoglycaemia and anoxia. A routine of soluble insulin injections with four-hourly testing of urine is the simplest, though wherever possible blood sugar estimations should be used. Although a test with Benedict solution is reliable, urine testing is now more usually and more easily performed with Clinitest tablets. The colour range is somewhat different but the interpretation is equally clear.

Colour Reaction of Urine to Clinitest		Dose of soluble insulin units
Blue	(0%)	No
Green (clear)	(0·25%)	Insulin
Turbid green	(0·50%)	
Brown/Green	(0·75%)	8–12
Yellow	(1%)	16
Orange	(2%+)	20

Four-hourly urine testing with periodic blood sugar estimations should be continued in the severe case for 48 hours post-operatively. The risk of infection, particularly pyelonephritis, discourages the use of a catheter left *in situ*, except where the patient is likely to remain unconscious for several days. Rough blood sugar estimations can be made on the spot using Dextrostix. These are accurate only in the lower ranges, so that they correctly indicate either hypoglycaemia or a normal blood sugar. They depend on a colour reaction of the sugar in a drop of capillary blood with a special reagent on the stick.

If in doubt, summon a physician.

Note.
(i) Post-operative coma is more likely to be caused by hypoglycaemia than hyperglycaemia if the above routine is performed. Give intravenous glucose and watch for the response.
(ii) Pre-operatively, never give oral glucose—it remains in

the stomach for a long time and is vomited again with depressing regularity.

(iii) Encourage your surgeon to place diabetic patients first on the morning operating list.

(iv) For emergencies, establish an intravenous infusion of glucose. Soluble insulin should be given subcutaneously, initially in a dose of 20 units for the first 50 g of glucose (1,000 ml of 5 per cent dextrose in water). This may need to be repeated in long operations or where return to oral feeding is delayed.

(6) There are an increasing number of drugs administered for medical reasons which affect the behaviour of anaesthetic drugs and therefore the course of anaesthesia. Some of these are listed below, and if you become a house-surgeon you will know what to ask, and record in your notes for the benefit of your anaesthetist, when a patient is admitted.

   (i) Many patients are on steroids these days. A simple preparation for surgery consists of maintaining the patient's normal steroid up to the operation and then giving 100 mg hydrocortisone intramuscularly at the time of premedication. This dose is repeated some eight to ten hours later, with a return to the patient's normal dosage as soon as possible thereafter. Occasionally, the administration of hydrocortisone in addition to the normal dosage must be continued and then gradually reduced over a period of two to three days. If exceptionally high doses of steroids have to be maintained for more than four days post-operatively, the risk of infection is increased and an antibiotic must be prescribed. In major operations, a fall in blood pressure indicates that the anaesthetist must inject a further dose of 100 mg hydrocortisone at once.

     These precautions apply not only to patients receiving steroids at the time of operation, but also to any who have undergone full-scale steroid therapy recently. Although active treatment may not be needed in all cases, those who have received steroids during the preceding two years must be observed with care. Patients who have received short periods of treatment with skin preparations or eye drops need no special treatment.

  (ii) Antihypertensive drugs such as reserpine, guanethidine, and methyldopa. These tend to cause a labile blood pressure, which can fall precipitously with haemorrhage or overshoot with the administration of the appropriate vasopressor. Nevertheless, treated hypertension is preferable to untreated. Although the effects of the above drugs can persist for two weeks or so after being withheld, a hypertensive crisis might occur without medication. When extensive surgery is contemplated, a short-acting antihypertensive agent might be substituted, but the patient will require supervision, possibly in hospital.

(iii) Phenothiazine drugs administered in large doses over a long period (to psychiatric patients) may provoke hypertension and prolonged unconsciousness.

(iv) Antibiotics (neomycin, polymyxin, and streptomycin have been implicated) in large doses can have a curariform action.

(v) Pitocin may cause cardiac irregularities under cyclopropane anaesthesia. It can also modify the action of scoline, producing an abnormal type of block of slow onset and long duration, but which may be reversed by neostigmine.

(vi) A massive blood transfusion can lead to "citrate intoxication" and the onset of cardiac failure. The mechanism is obscure, and probably only occurs in individuals with seriously damaged livers (where citrate is normally broken down). Of greater significance may be the liberation of large amounts of free potassium present in stored blood, in which the pH falls progressively and can produce a metabolic acidosis. Although most of the citrate is rapidly broken down into water and carbon dioxide, some combines with calcium and is excreted as calcium citrate. Thus there could be an ionic imbalance due to loss of calcium, aggravated by the excess potassium. The administration of 1 g of calcium gluconate should therefore accompany large, rapidly administered transfusions in patients with hepatic disease.

(vii) Sedatives and analgesics will have the same action as heavy premedication.

(viii) More and more patients are receiving monoamine oxidase inhibitors for mild psychiatric disorders. In such patients vasopressors and pethidine should be avoided.

(ix) Long term anticoagulant therapy (usually with warfarin) after a coronary thrombosis can make surgery hazardous. For the anaesthetist, most forms of local

analgesia are contraindicated by the risk of haemorrhage. For the same reason, endotracheal intubation
must be performed most carefully.

(x) Treatment with ecothiopate (Phospholine iodide),
which is a long-acting anticholinesterase may be
encountered in an eye department. Prolonged paralysis
may follow the administration of a muscle relaxant,
especially suxemethonium, in such patients.

Considerations Concerning the Operation

Divide all your cases into:

(1) Those requiring profound muscular relaxation.
(2) Those not requiring profound muscular relaxation.

The former category is filled almost entirely by abdominal
operations, those on the upper abdomen calling for a deeper
level of anaesthesia than those on the lower. Gynaecology
requires deep anaesthesia or curarization owing to the fondness
of its practitioners for wide incisions and slight respiratory
movement.

For all anaesthetists, experienced or otherwise, *emergency
abdominal operations* present a special difficulty — the risk of
active vomiting, or the equally sinister passive regurgitation.
These must always be remembered as serious possibilities. If
your competence permits the passage of a cuffed endotracheal
tube, then anaesthesia may be induced with thiopentone and
suxemethonium while an assistant applies pressure to the
cricothyroid ring to compress the oesophagus. The patient must
first breathe oxygen for 2–3 minutes so that no time need be
lost between the injection and the placing of the endotracheal
tube. Alternatively, a stomach tube may be passed pre-
operatively (but remember that regardless of size, it cannot
cope with solid fish and chips) or anaesthesia may be induced
in the left lateral position.

Despite these measures, watch carefully for regurgitation
from the stomach. If it occurs, tilt the patient's head down and
attend to the pharynx with a sucker, as advised on page 27. An
intravenous infusion should be established before taking the
patient into the theatre.

Ophthalmic, orthopaedic, and E.N.T. surgery may be
accomplished under light anaesthesia. The operation of dissection tonsillectomy is best performed in an adult with a nasal
endotracheal tube *in situ*, but children should be given benefit
of the *Boyle-Davis gag*. The secret of the successful use of this

piece of apparatus lies in bringing the patient to a reasonably deep state of anaesthesia first, insufflating about 10 litres a minute of a mixture of gas, oxygen, and ether or halothane (2%) through the delivery pipe, and employing an efficient suction pump to clear the blood away from the pharynx. All E.N.T. patients that have not, unfortunately, recovered their cough reflex by the end of the operation must be positioned and otherwise guarded against the inhalation of blood.

Obstetrics

Obstetrics is a controversial subject and so is anaesthetics. Where the two meet, therefore, a lively disagreement on technique may be expected. The following suggestions may nevertheless be helpful to the student.

(1) **Analgesia.** In this country, the relief of pain during labour is often achieved by a method of self-administration by the mother under the supervision of a midwife. The techniques in common use seek to provide the maximum comfort for the mother without depressing the foetus. Such a compromise is effected by a combination of methods:
  (i) The administration of a continuously acting drug like pethidine or morphine, and
  (ii) the intermittent inhalation of a weak anaesthetic mixture (nitrous oxide or trichlorethylene) when uterine contractions are painful.

It is unusual for either (i) or (ii) to be sufficient by themselves, but together they can produce effective control of pain, provided:
  (i) the mother realizes the implication of analgesia (relief of pain without loss of all sensation)
  (ii) the attendant is similarly well educated
  (iii) analgesia is started early enough in labour
  (iv) the mother learns to breathe from her apparatus when the uterus begins to contract — not when she feels pain
  (v) the apparatus is working correctly
  (vi) the labour is normal
  (vii) the attendant is not hardened by familiarity to a state of indifference to the sensations of the mother.

No mixture which might cause asphyxia in the mother and consequent oxygen lack in the foetus can be tolerated.

Premixed nitrous oxide and oxygen in the proportions of

50:50 in a single cylinder is now widely available, and provides a constant predictable gas mixture which ensures adequate oxygenation. The apparatus requires little more than a demand valve attached to the cylinder, making a relatively simple, foolproof device. The Entonox apparatus (as the above is known) has Central Midwives Board approval, and has achieved even wider use in a variety of circumstances where pain relief is required (e.g., by ambulance crews at the scene of road accidents).

Because of its high analgesic property, trichlorethylene has proved highly effective in obstetrics. Two trichlorethylene inhalers have been approved for use by midwives. These machines, the Tecota and the Emotril, deliver a constant 0·5% concentration of trichlorethylene in air under all conditions. In addition, methoxyflurane — a highly effective analgesic — has achieved some popularity and has received the seal of approval of the Central Midwives Board. It may be conveniently administered from a Cardiff inhaler, which delivers 0·35% in air.

All these inhalers, which are connected to the patient by a wide-bore corrugated hose, expiratory valve, and mask, have an air-vent near the face-piece as an additional safeguard. Once the unconscious patient's finger relaxes its pressure on the vent, only air is breathed from the machine.

In hospital practice a wider range of analgesics may be used, and these include continuous caudal or extradural block (see p. 121). These methods are increasingly popular, the lumbar approach gaining in favour because the needle and catheter is further removed from possible contamination with urine or faeces. Lumbar analgesia is somewhat more controllable, though undoubtedly the caudal approach is safer in unskilled hands. The performance and supervision of either require considerable skill and judgement, which limits their use despite their offering the most effective pain relief available. From a practical standpoint, it is now accepted that suitably trained midwives may administer "top-up" doses on the written instructions of a doctor.

Some obstetricians favour the use of a mixture of pethidine and levallorphan (Pethilorfan) as an alternative to pethidine to avoid depression of the foetus, but it is of questionable practical value. Phenothiazine drugs also have found some favour, but their use is restricted to patients needing general sedation (e.g., pre-eclampsia) rather than pain relief. Midwives are not allowed to use these drugs.

(2) **Normal delivery.** Apart from the analgesia which may be provided during the course of labour, it may be necessary to provide anaesthesia for the delivery itself. As a rule, this is needed only for the crowning of the head and the delivery of the head and shoulders, but on occasions the anaesthetic may have to be protracted to allow the performance of an episiotomy, the delivery, and the repair of the episiotomy. Often, efficient general analgesia (with nitrous oxide or trichlorethylene) and a pudendal block will be adequate. If not, a full nitrous-oxide anaesthesia with or without supplementation by trichlorethylene or ether will be best.

(3) **Caesarean section.** A simple technique may be employed with great success, despite the standing controversy on the anaesthesia for this operation. Gas, oxygen, and trichlorethylene followed by gas, oxygen, and ether, an abundance of oxygen being administered, is entirely satisfactory if one observes:

(i) No morphine in the premedication. Atropine 0·6 mg only should be administered. Thiopentone may be used for induction if a dose just sufficient to bring about unconsciousness is given (never more than 0·25 g).

(ii) The abdomen is already stretched, so little anaesthetic need be administered. Satisfactory relaxation is present even if the mother's feet have to be restrained against reflex movement following the initial incision. Once the umbilical cord is divided the narcosis may be made as deep as desired.

(iii) An excess of oxygen should be administered until the baby is born.

(iv) Halothane may be substituted for trichlorethylene to assist induction. Note well though: halothane relaxes the uterus and must be used only in minimal quantities and only for induction, or there may be serious haemorrhage. This applies to forceps delivery as well.

(v) There is all the difference in the world between an emergency and an elective Caesarean section. The former demands all the safeguards afforded a patient for an emergency abdominal operation (p. 129).

(vi) The expert would probably recommend nitrous oxide and oxygen with a muscle relaxant as less likely to depress the foetus. Our comments about this sequence of agents apply equally forcibly here as in other situations.

(4) **Forceps delivery.** This may be undertaken under light anaesthesia with nitrous oxide and oxygen combined with trichlorethylene or ether.

Beware in obstetric practice of vomiting during induction, resulting from an unavoidable unpreparedness of the mother. Remember also the risk of regurgitation (see p. 105).

Obstetric patients not in labour, but requiring an anaesthetic, are not such difficult problems. The patient may be prepared in the usual way, and deep anaesthesia does not affect the foetus. Any patient is open to the usual surgical emergencies, but these remarks apply to such procedures as examination under anaesthesia, artificial rupture of the membranes, and external version. Remember that all patients with large abdominal tumours, of which full-term, pregnant women are prime examples, may have difficulty in breathing (splinting of diaphragm). The tumour may press and occlude the inferior vena cava. Circulatory collapse follows rapidly, reversed by turning the patient on her side.

Neonatal Resuscitation

After an operative delivery, whether by forceps or Caesarean section, there may be difficulty in establishing the baby's respiration. This may be caused by respiratory depression following the anaesthetic or other depressant drugs given to the mother, or by the obstetrical complications making such a delivery necessary. Time should not be wasted in academic discussions about the cause of the trouble. Though the foetus is surprisingly resistant to oxygen lack and carbon dioxide excess, permanent damage will inevitably follow unless treatment is instituted.

The degree of respiratory depression may be gauged from the baby's colour, pulse, muscle tone, attempts at breathing, and reflex activity. These signs may be helpful in assessing the success or otherwise of your treatment, which should consist of:

(1) Clear mucus or meconium from the nose, mouth, and pharynx of the baby.

(2) Apply a mild stimulus, such as slapping the soles of the feet.

(3) Apply a face mask delivering oxygen.

(4) If there is no improvement — and not more than two minutes should be spent on the foregoing — the infant should be intubated with the smallest size tube available

and the lungs inflated with oxygen (limiting the pressure to 25 cm H_2O). In an emergency, mouth to mouth respiration should be used.

(5) If there is reason to believe that the foetal depression is caused by pethidine given to the mother, administer levallorphan 0·25 mg via the umbilical vein.

(6) The administration of other drugs via the umbilical vein is of dubious value and may cause more harm than good.

(7) Like a good Boy Scout, Be Prepared — this situation can arise after *any* delivery.

CHAPTER 13

How To Give An Anaesthetic

Finally, a summary to correlate much of the information previously given — how to administer a straightforward anaesthetic.

The patient has been examined, the premedication given, and the anaesthetic decided upon. The anaesthetist is ready in the anaesthetic room, and has not omitted to wash his hands before approaching his patient.

(1) **Check the apparatus,** and wash it through with gas to eliminate any irritant vapour collected therein.

(2) **Induction**
(i) With thiopentone. Inject sufficient thiopentone to bring the patient to the stage of light surgical anaesthesia, as described in Chapter 5. Gently elicit the eyelash reflex if in doubt.

(ii) With nitrous oxide. Hold the mask a few inches above the face, and allow the gas to run down on to the patient's nose and mouth, the while carrying on a soothing and reassuring monologue. Continue until the respiration is regular.

(3) **Continuing induction,** after either (i) or (ii) above.
(i) Apply the mask to the face with the right hand, maintaining an air-tight fit and holding the chin forward. The function of this hand during induction is as important as that of the left, which is free to manipulate the machine.

(ii) Turn down the nitrous oxide to 6 litres/minute and turn the oxygen up to 2 litres/minute. Move the control of the vaporizer (trichlorethylene or halothane) to ''just on'' — equivalent probably to rather less than 0.5%.

(iii) Thereafter increase the vapour strength by advancing the control slightly after every two or three breaths until 1% trichlorethylene (or about 2% halothane) is being delivered.

134

Watch the reservoir bag, which should be comfortably full. If it is not, there must be a leak in the circuit allowing the admission of air to dilute the mixture.

(iv) Coughing or breath holding requires a halt to be made in the advancement of the control.

(v) Once the patient has settled a change may be made to ether if desired. By this time the patient should be deep enough to tolerate an airway, after which the mask may be strapped on with a harness, and the trolley taken into the theatre.

(4) **In the theatre** be sure the patient is placed on the table without danger of incurring a palsy — the radial and median nerves are the most vulnerable. See that the hands are secure but not undergoing pressure, and that the heels are not overlapping the table. No part of the patient must be touching bare metal lest a contact be made if the surgeon uses the diathermy, followed by a burn and an action for damages. There is growing recognition of the hazards from the increased use of electronic monitoring, and concern about the electrical safety of these devices. When two or more are attached to a patient the danger arises of an abnormal current flow, which could lead to burns or even ventricular fibrillation. Advice should be sought whenever there is doubt about the compatibility of these machines, especially when surgical diathermy is employed (this provides a high intensity current which may, in some circumstances, not escape through the usual, large indifferent electrode). The risks occur not only in the operating theatre but in the recovery room and intensive care unit as well.

As soon as the patient is settled on the table check the oxygen supply and take the patient's pulse. A knowledge of the initial pulse rate is essential for judgment of the patient's later condition. In major surgery, observation of the blood pressure also is advisable.

The depth of anaesthesia must be increased if an abdominal operation is proposed, as described on p. 55. Alternatively, the desired condition can be obtained by the use of a muscle relaxant, maintaining light anaesthesia throughout.

During the operation there are six objects for your close attention:

(i) The reservoir bag. This reveals:
  (*a*) whether the patient is breathing at all.
  (*b*) whether he is too light or too deep (see p. 29).
  (*c*) after a little practice, the intermediate planes of narcosis.

(ii) The patient's colour (see pp. 30, 81).
(iii) The patient's pulse (see p. 81).
(iv) The progress of the operation, including the amount of blood being lost.
(v) The type of the patient's respiration and other signs to determine the depth of the anaesthesia (see p. 37).
    Train yourself to interpret these signs at all operations to achieve proficiency.
(vi) An occasional check on the quantity of the liquid anaesthetic remaining, and of the amount and flow rate of the gases.
(vii) And you must *keep up the patient's chin*, unless an endotracheal tube is in place.

(5) **Towards the end of the operation** (at the closure of the peritoneum in abdominal cases) the anaesthetic should be lightened or discontinued altogether. If a muscle relaxant is used, artificial ventilation will have to be performed throughout the operation. The effects of any relaxant must be reversed (p. 56) and the anaesthetist must be satisfied that normal, spontaneous respiration has returned before handing over the patient. Except in very exceptional circumstances (e.g., after some plastic or orthopaedic procedures when changes in posture are impossible) the patient should be placed on his side. This does not release the nurse from the obligation of maintaining support to the chin until she is satisfied that the airway is satisfactory and/or the patient has recovered consciousness.

Medico-Legal

The anaesthetist is particularly liable to litigation because the consequences of his errors are likely to be quickly apparent. But his standards of conduct and practice are no different from those required of all other doctors. Any blame must be related to his seniority, and to his performance of acts which are considered to be accepted practice. *Res ipsa loquitur*[1] is no longer an inviolate argument. Negligence must be proved. So the anaesthetist who works within his capabilities and uses methods generally considered safe and reasonable has nothing to fear. But certain safeguards must be adopted.

(1) Check and double check the identity of the patient, the operation to be performed, and the side to be operated on before starting the anaesthetic.

[1] Legal Latin, meaning "It's bloody obvious".

(2) See that the patient has signed the standard form of consent approved by the protection societies and the DHSS. If the patient is under sixteen, it must be signed by his parent or guardian. The senile and the insane need the consent of a relative or someone responsible for them. Special consent is needed for sterilization and termination of pregnancy. Remember that Jehovah's Witnesses refuse blood transfusions. Consent is valid in law only if given without duress and without the influence of drugs — the anaesthetic room is not the right place to ask a premedicated patient to sign a legal document.

(3) Check all drugs and apparatus personally. This includes diathermy and electrical connections (see p. 136).

(4) Check any blood to be administered most carefully (see p. 87).

(5) Never start an anaesthetic unless a third person is present. Apart from the need of help if difficulties arise, dreaming under light anaesthesia is not uncommon and can lead to complaints of sexual assault.

(6) Be guarded in conversation during induction and recovery from anaesthesia. Misunderstandings at such times are common.

(7) Check the position of a patient on the operating table and post-operatively on the trolley or in bed to avoid injury.

(8) Always fill in an anaesthetic record card.

(9) In the event of a mishap, write detailed notes as soon as possible and keep these carefully.

(10) Deaths within twenty-four hours of an operation must be reported to the coroner. The report (the nature of which varies from place to place) on the events leading to death must be submitted as soon as possible.

(11) To be employed in the National Health Service you must be a member of one of the defence societies. Inform them immediately of any untoward incident and send a detailed report. This is not a responsibility of the student, who cannot become a member of a society until he is medically qualified.

(12) Honesty is essential between you and your legal advisers. Discussion, or imparting information about any incident, with the patient, relatives or friends is the responsibility of a qualified doctor. The student should take no part in these.

Much of this reads like more repetition of advice given in earlier pages. So it is. But unless you can satisfy yourself, and other people too, on these points, you will find yourself on shaky legal ground, as well as behaving quite indefensibly in the clinical care of your patient.

Last Word

You are probably now too frightened to approach an anaesthetic machine. If so, this pamphlet has not failed in its object, for a knowledge of the possible dangers associated with anaesthesia is essential to ensure a safe administration.

The emergencies of the subject have been treated with emphasis, but none should arise in a thoughtful and careful administration. Remember the best way to get out of trouble is to avoid it, and observe at all times *safety first*. Common sense is the basis of good anaesthesia — but then, so is it the foundation of all medicine.

INDEX